Diet only two days a week. The weight-loss and healthy living plan that anyone can do

This small book provide[s] [...] [follo]wing the 5:2 diet, written in an easy-to-fo[llow and friendly] style by Jacqueline Whitehart. Jacqueline was o[ne of the] first followers of what is now known as the 5:2 diet. She continues to follow the diet and is one of its most well-regarded advocates.

This practical book gives you all the advice and tips you need to get started on this diet. There's week-by-week updates on what and when you should eat. Plus tips and motivation right when you need it.

Jacqueline has devised a full range of over 100 fantastic, filling recipes, from breakfasts to snacks, light lunches and dinners. The recipes are expertly balanced with plenty of protein and moderate complex carbohydrates. They're all designed to fill you up and stave off hunger pangs.

The 5:2 diet has a simple basis. 2 days per week you eat a quarter of your normal recommended calories – that's 500 for women and 650 for men. These are your fasting days. The other 5 days are feast days, when you can eat what you want. Sounds easy? That's because it is.

Read on to get started on a healthier, lighter future.

Brand new recipes, exercises and chat all available on my website

www.52recipes.co.uk

Important note

The information and advice contained in this book are intended as a general guide to dieting and healthy eating and are not specific to individuals or their particular circumstances. This book is not intended to replace treatment by a qualified practitioner. Neither the authors nor the publishers can be held responsible for claims arising from inappropriate use of any dietary regime. Do not attempt self-diagnosis or self-treatment for serious or long-term conditions without consulting a medical professional or qualified practitioner.

First published in Great Britain in 2012 by **Pepik Ltd**. First published in the United States in 2013 by **Pepik Ltd**.

enquiries@pepikbooks.com

www.pepikbooks.com

Table of Contents

Introduction

For two non-consecutive days each week you follow a restricted calorie diet – that's 500 calories for women and 650 for men. The other five days a week you eat whatever you like.

As well as being an excellent way to lose weight the long-term health benefits of this diet are impressive. Following the 5:2 diet can reduce cholesterol levels, cut your risk of diabetes, lower your cancer risk and delay the onset of Alzheimer's. Find out the latest research results in the "How the 5:2 diet can help you live longer" chapter of this book.

I may be an expert dieter but I am definitely not a scientist so I have chosen to concentrate on the weight-loss element of the diet. You shouldn't forget that by following the 5:2 diet you may well be extending your good health for longer into old age.

As with all diets you should seek advice from a health professional before starting. This is especially true if you have any particular health concerns. This diet is definitely **not** recommended if you are pregnant or breast-feeding, diabetic or hypoglycemic.

As a typical working mom I've always found a lack of time and motivation for diets. They just simply don't fit in with a busy lifestyle, my love of potato chips, and the desire for a glass of wine after a hard day wrangling kids. So I've tried many things: the Atkins diet, calorie counting, and gym membership, to name only three. They all start off well and then slowly fade away as other things in life take priority.

But the 5:2 diet has been different. I came across the diet quite by chance and was so impressed by the claimed health benefits that I decided it was worth a try. The weight-loss element of the diet was just one of the aspects that appealed.

Straight away I saw the benefits. Immediate weight-loss and increased energy. After only a week the fasting days became simple and easy to slot into my lifestyle. Now they hold no fear and I even find myself looking forward to them. I love the fact that for most of the week I can eat what I want and not worry about it.

Quite simply this diet has changed my life so much and given me so many benefits that I have, for the first time in my life, felt the need to share this breakthrough diet with as many people as possible. I hope it works as well for you as it has for me.

Special thanks must go to Katie Buffalo who has helped me enormously in adapting the recipes for the American market. You wouldn't be reading this without her invaluable assistance.

If you like this book then please take a look at my new book, The 5:2 Bikini Diet. 140 delicious recipes for summer and an exclusive exercise plan to get you beach ready. Available on amazon.com.

Yours,

Jacqueline

Jacqueline Whitehart

Why the 5:2 diet?

The 5:2 diet is for you, for me, for everyone. It's proven to be easier to stick to than other diets. Why? Because its rules are so simple AND because you only diet two days a week. For five full days you are not on a diet. Because you know that following each day on which you diet you can eat normally the motivation to complete the diet day without giving in to temptation is high. And when you see yourself losing weight and still continuing to eat as normal 5 days a week it's easy to find the strength to carry on.

With the 5:2 diet you really can "**eat cake and lose weight too**".

There are three main benefits of the 5:2 diet. The first is of course losing weight, which is done gradually and safely, meaning the pounds stay off for good.

The second is that it is easy to follow and stick to; in fact, early stages of research into comparisons between this diet and others show that after a six week period a significantly higher proportion of 5:2 dieters were sticking to the diet than any other weight-loss plan. It is the knowledge that you only ever have to wait until the next morning that makes it so easy to keep going. It certainly works for me: I always look forward to my breakfast on the evening of my diet day, imagining the delights I can eat. But the strange thing is, when I wake up the next morning I'm not even particularly hungry.

The third is the most amazing health benefits that this simple diet seems to offer. It seems that the 5:2 diet can reduce the risks of some of the diseases we associate with aging; in particular heart disease, some cancers and Alzheimer's. Because the effects of intermittent fasting, of which the 5:2 diet is one variant, have not been fully researched long-term we can't state or prove all of these benefits, but all the research done so far on the 5:2 (and other very similar diets such as Intermittent Fasting (IF), Alternate Day Fasting (ADF) and the Two-day diet) show promising results. Take a look at the chapter "How the 5:2 diet can help you live longer" if you want to find out about the existing research in more detail.

The 5:2 diet and me

Before I started the 5:2 diet I weighed in at 153 pounds, size 12, with a BMI of 23.4. Not in the overweight category, but slowly and inexorably creeping towards it. Before I had children I was always around 140 pounds but by the time I'd had my third child I found it close to impossible to shift the excess weight.

Four months after starting the 5:2 diet I was 142 pounds. I am now a much happier size 8 with a BMI of 21.6.

Since then I've maintained my weight at approximately that level through fasting one or two days a week. I continue to eat healthily but without dieting on the other days.

Before I started this diet I thought I suffered with low blood sugar; I could never skip a meal and by lunchtime I would always be starving and grumpy. Within a couple of weeks of following the 5:2 diet I had noticed a huge difference. I follow Plan 1 for women, allowing myself a small snack for lunch and more often than not a stew and some green vegetables for my dinner (as this is something my whole family can enjoy). I've included all my favorites in the recipe section.

Getting started

There's no time like the present to get started with the 5:2 diet. If you are healthy and do not have any medical conditions such as diabetes then you are ready to go.

The principle rules of 5:2 dieting are simple. Twice a week you follow a calorie-restricted diet (500 calories for women and 650 for men) while the rest of the week you can eat whatever you like.

On your diet days you are shocking your body into breaking down more fat. On your non-diet days you eat what you want but it is virtually impossible to make up the missing calories. Research has shown that an average person eats at most 10-15% more than normal on the day following a diet day.

What's more it's incredibly simple to do. Once you get over some hunger pangs in the first week or two your body adapts to the restricted calories on your diet days, meaning the 5:2 diet is extremely easy to stick to in the long-term.

In this book I'll guide and encourage you through every step of the first few weeks. With menu plans and scrumptious recipe ideas you'll find the 5:2 diet easy to follow and stick with. So let's get started and plan your first day.

Choosing your diet days

At the start of each week you should see what days would fit in best with your schedule. Remember the days need to be non-consecutive. Obviously days where you have social arrangements, or when you plan to eat out or have drinks with friends, should not be diet days. You should see this as one of the great advantages of this plan. You can still enjoy going out to restaurants, eating desserts guilt-free and generally enjoying life as it should be enjoyed.

For your fasting days you should choose the least social days on your calendar. They are likely to be work days – work is a great distraction from food – and days when you have plenty going on.

The only restriction on your diet days is that you must have a rest day between fasts. The diet days can change each week – making it the ultimate flexible diet. You just need to check off two days each week as diet days and you will be right on track to some impressive health and weight-loss benefits.

In the first two weeks of the diet your diet days should also be relatively quiet days. Days when you don't have important meetings, are not doing anything too physical and when you are not likely to be exposed to a lot of nice food and cooking. This is because in the first 2 weeks of the diet you may suffer from hunger pangs, feel slightly light-headed at times and generally be in need of a spot of will-power. But you can be sure as each fasting day is completed successfully the next will be significantly easier. By week three diet days should become an easy and regular part of your routine, not holding you back at all.

When to eat, What to eat

Before you start on your first diet day it is wise to think about how best to manage your food over the day. To do this you need to think about your lifestyle and your body's needs. Here are a few questions that might help you decide what and when to eat.

- Are you working in an office?
- Are you busy during the day with little time to think about food?
- Are you time pressed so cooking is difficult?
- Are you exposed to unhealthy food during the day?
- Are you cranky if you miss breakfast?
- Do you feel most hungry in the evenings?
- When do you tend to get food cravings?

There are various ways in which to split your calories throughout the day; each one will be described in detail shortly. But as a general guide if you tend to be super busy during the day with no time to stop you should go for a breakfast and dinner option. But if you're in a rush in the morning and aren't particularly hungry first thing you should try an option with more food at lunch and dinner-time.

Menu planning

Here we must split into different plans for men and women. As men are allowed 650 calories on their diet days (compared to 500 calories for women) they have more options for what and when to eat. Don't worry ladies, they are not going to feel any less hungry than you.

Menu plans for women

Plan 1 (no breakfast)

Breakfast: 2 cups tea or coffee with skim milk or sugar free, fat free creamer OR 1/2 cup of skim or soy milk

-

Lunch: light lunch or snack, totaling 150 calories

-

Dinner: main meal, totaling 300 calories

Plan 2 (no lunch)

Breakfast: up to 200 calories, including beverages

-

Lunch: NO LUNCH

-

Dinner: main meal, totaling 300 calories

Plan 3 (3 small meals)

Breakfast: up to 150 calories, including beverages

-

Lunch: up to 150 calories

-

Dinner: up to 200 calories

Ladies, you should choose which of these plans works for you best, or make up your own! Try it out using the detailed menu plans on the following pages for each option. All of the recipes are designed to be healthy and filling, helping you to stave off those hunger pangs.

If this looks scary or difficult, it's not – I, Jacqueline Whitehart, hater of diets with a shortage of will-power, totally promise! Your body soon adapts to the lower amount of calories and you definitely won't starve. Above all, remember that your reward is to eat what you want tomorrow AND still watch the weight fall off.

Menu plans for men

Plan A (no breakfast)

Breakfast: 2 cups tea or coffee with skim milk or sugar free, fat free creamer OR ½ cup of skim or soy milk.

\-

Lunch: up to 300 calories

\-

Dinner: main meal, totaling 300 calories

Plan B (no lunch)

Breakfast: full breakfast, totaling up to 300 calories

\-

Lunch: tiny snack (50 calories)

\-

Dinner: main meal, totaling 300 calories

Plan C (3 small meals)

Breakfast: up to 150 calories, including beverages

\-

Lunch: 200 calories

\-

Dinner: main meal, totaling 300 calories

Following the menu planners

These menu planners have been put together based on the recipes in this book. The recipes have all been designed to be healthy, to fill you up and to stave off hunger pangs. The recipes are high in protein and complex carbohydrates, while being low in fat. Some are designed to be prepared quickly and easily for one, others are designed to be cooked in bigger portions and either shared with the family or frozen in individual servings (practically all of the recipes here are freezer-friendly) so you have a perfect ready-to-eat meal in minutes without resorting to low-cal TV dinners.

Speaking of TV dinners, they do have a place in this diet – and they're great to have around for those times you want to skip cooking altogether. Lean Cuisine and Healthy Choice brand frozen meals are available everywhere and they are almost all between 200-300 calories – and some of them, especially those with lots of veggies, aren't that bad!

For men, this means that you could have frozen meals for lunch and dinner, (as long as both are under 300 calories and you've just had tea or coffee for breakfast).

For women, you could have a Lean Cuisine entree for lunch (under 300 calories), or swap your lunch and dinner and have a frozen meal for lunch followed by a light snack in the evening.

Please remember that while frozen meals are an ideal quick fix, they are expensive and NOTHING beats home cooking for a nutritious filling meal. The recipes in this book are designed to give you a great balance of protein and carbohydrates.

Menu plan 1 (for women, no breakfast)

Breakfast is strictly limited to 2 cups of tea or coffee made with skim milk or sugar-free, fat-free creamer OR one latte coffee made with skim milk (see recipes) OR ½ cup of skim milk. Total calories should be less than fifty for breakfast.

Week 1

	Lunch	Dinner	Cals
Day 1	Smoked salmon and cream cheese on Crispbread **page 56** *169 cals*	Chicken with orange and black olives, **page 98** *284 cals*	453
Day 2	Spicy butternut squash soup, **page 74** *169 cals*	Scallops with garlic tomatoes, **page 109** *258 cals*	427

Week 2

	Lunch	Dinner	Cals
Day 1	Savoy cabbage and bacon soup, **page 71** *156 cals*	Steak in mushrooms and wine, **page 128** *294 cals*	450
Day 2	Oriental shrimp and mushroom salad, **page 47** *151 cals*	Sticky Thai chicken with 2 new potatoes and broccoli, **page 94** *305 cals*	456

Week 3

	Lunch	Dinner	Cals
Day 1	Pastrami on RyKrisp, **page 54** *137 cals*	Sweet potato chili with 25g white rice, **page 87** *300 cals*	437
Day 2	Italian bread salad, **page 48** *170 cals*	Chunky cod with tomatoes and spinach, **page 107** *248 cals*	418

Menu plan 2 (for women, no lunch)

The total calories per day on this plan add up to approximately 450 calories. This is to allow for 2 cups of tea or coffee with milk OR a tiny snack (e.g. a piece of fruit) at lunch.

Week 1

	Breakfast	Dinner	Cals
Day 1	Breakfast Burrito, **page 42** *185 cals*	Chunky cod with tomatoes and spinach, **page 107** *248 cals*	**433**
Day 2	Ham omelet, **page 58** *198 cals*	One pot Vegetable Tagine, **page 90** *247 cals*	**445**

Week 2

	Breakfast	Dinner	Cals
Day 1	"Fast" Food breakfast sandwich **page 41** *197 cals*	Quick fried steak with salsa verde, **page 124** served with 1 cup green beans (35 cals) *259 cals*	**456**
Day 2	Oatmeal pot, **page 40** and an apple (53 cals) *179 cals*	Chicken in tomato sauce, **page 96** served with 1 cup broccoli (33 cals) *288 cals*	**467**

Week 3

	Breakfast	Dinner	Cals
Day 1	Home-made Granola, **page 43** made with ½ cup skim milk *199 cals*	Honey Mustard Pork Chop, **page 121** served with ½ cup curly kale (16 cals) *234 cals*	**433**
Day 2	Breakfast Burrito, **page 42** *185 cals*	Salmon and cod fishcakes, **page 108** *256 cals*	**441**

Menu plan 3 (for women, 3 small meals)

Week 1

	Breakfast	Lunch	Dinner	Cals
Day 1	Natural yogurt with blueberries **page 39** *91 cals*	Oriental shrimp and mushroom salad, **page 47** *151 cals*	Ramen soup with udon noodles, **page 77** *215 cals*	**457**
Day 2	Egg white omelet, **page 38** *57 cals*	Lentil, lemon and thyme soup, **page 69** *121 cals*	Creamy chicken curry, **page 95** with ¼ cup white rice (70 cals) *315 cals*	**493**

Week 2

	Breakfast	Lunch	Dinner	Cals
Day 1	Oatmeal pot **page 40** and an apple (53 cals) *179 cals*	Chargrilled vegetable salad, **page 46** *127 cals*	Portobello mushrooms with spinach and tomato, **page 86** *195 cals*	**501**
Day 2	Blackberry fool, **page 38** *45 cals*	Pastrami on RyKrisp, **page 54** *137 cals*	Autumn lamb stew **page 119** with 2 new potatoes and ¼ cup peas *320 cals*	**502**

Week 3

	Breakfast	Lunch	Dinner	Cals
Day 1	Hot chocolate, **page 39** *102 cals*	Crispbread with peanut butter and tomato, **page 54** *97 cals*	Quick fried steak with Salsa Verde, **page 124** served with ½ cup green beans (35 cals) *259 cals*	**458**
Day 2	Egg white omelet, **page 38** *57 cals*	Spicy butternut squash soup, **page 74** *169 cals*	Scallops with garlic tomatoes, **page 109** *258 cals*	**484**

Menu plan A (for men, no breakfast)

Breakfast is strictly limited to 2 cups of tea or coffee made with skim milk or sugar-free, fat-free creamer OR one latte coffee made with skim milk (see recipes) OR a ½ cup glass of skim milk. Total calories should be less than fifty for breakfast.

Week 1			
	Lunch	**Dinner**	**Cals**
Day 1	Hearty ham soup, **page 78** *224 cals*	Tilapia with a herb crust, **page 104** with 4 new potatoes and ½ cup spinach *334 cals*	558
Day 2	Roast chicken and pesto open flatbread, **page 61** *241 cals*	Chili con carne, **page 126** with ½ cup white rice *365 cals*	606
Week 2			
	Lunch	**Dinner**	**Cals**
Day 1	Refried beans and goat's cheese hot wrap, **page 59** *268 cals*	Steak in mushrooms and wine, **page 128** with 1 cup broccoli *327 cals*	595
Day 2	Ham omelet, **page 58** with half slice granary bread *298 cals*	Chunky cod with tomatoes and spinach, **page 107** with 2 new potatoes *318 cals*	616
Week 3			
	Lunch	**Dinner**	**Cals**
Day 1	Ramen soup with udon noodles, **page 77** *215 cals*	Creamy chicken curry, **page 95** with ½ cup white rice *376 cals*	591
Day 2	Two Open-faced BLTs, **page 57** *346 cals*	Steamed salmon with Chinese vegetables, **page 113** *296 cals*	642

Menu plan B (for men, no lunch)

Where half slice of bread is listed this could be a whole slice of
"diet" bread or ½ thick slice of whole wheat or whole grain bread.

Week 1

	Breakfast	Dinner	Cals
Day 1	Breakfast Burrito **page 42** with 1 tbsp grated cheddar *265 cals*	Fresh pesto cod, **page 105** with 4 new potatoes and ½ cup spinach *336 cals*	601
Day 2	Scrambled eggs with peppers and tomatoes, **page 44** *249 cals*	Chili con carne, **page 126** with ½ cup white rice *365 cals*	614

Week 2

	Breakfast	Dinner	Cals
Day 1	Double portion of Oatmeal pot, **page 40** *252 cals*	Chicken with Orange and black olives, **page 98** with 2 new potatoes and 1 cup broccoli *387 cals*	639
Day 2	Ham omelet, **page 58** with ½ slice wholegrain bread *298 cals*	Steamed salmon with Chinese vegetables, **page 113** *296 cals*	594

Week 3

	Breakfast	Dinner	Cals
Day 1	2 Open-face BLTs **page 57** *346 cals*	One pot Thai curry, **page 89** *242 cals*	588
Day 2	"Fast" food breakfast sandwich, **page 41** with small apple *278 cals*	Quick fried steak with Salsa Verde, **page 124** with 2 new potatoes and 1 cup green beans *327 cals*	605

Menu plan C (for men, 3 small meals)

Week 1

	Breakfast	Lunch	Dinner	Cals
Day 1	Natural yogurt with blueberries, **page 39** *91 cals*	Warm leek and lentil salad with goat's cheese, **page 52** *298 cals*	Honey Mustard pork chop, **page 121** with 1 cup broccoli *251 cals*	640
Day 2	"Fast" Food Breakfast Sandwich, **page 41** *197cals*	Shrimp in sweet chili sauce wrap, **page 61** *239 cals*	Portobello mushrooms with spinach and tomato, **page 86** *195 cals*	631

Week 2

	Breakfast	Lunch	Dinner	Cals
Day 1	Breakfast Burrito, **page 42** *185 cals*	Chargrilled vegetable salad, **page 46** *127 cals*	Paprika pork casserole, **page 129** with ½ cup spinach *319 cals*	631
Day 2	Oatmeal pot, **page 40** *126 cals*	Smoked salmon with cucumber on crispbread, **page 56** *195 cals*	Chicken with brown mushrooms, **page 97** with ½ cup kale *300 cals*	621

Week 3

	Breakfast	Lunch	Dinner	Cals
Day 1	Scrambled eggs with peppers and tomatoes, **page 44** *249 cals*	Ham or bacon salad, **page 46** *98 cals*	Scallops with garlic tomatoes, **page 109** *258 cals*	605
Day 2	Hot chocolate, **page 39** *102 cals*	Refried beans and goat's cheese hot wrap, **page 59** *268 cals*	Quick fried steak with Salsa Verde, **page 124** with 1 cup green beans *259 cals*	629

Frequently Asked Questions

Q: Can I have caffeinated beverages?

A: Yes

Do you drink coffee or tea or colas regularly every day? You are definitely not alone. I do NOT advise you to give them up, even on your diet days. Why? Because caffeine withdrawal is likely to give you headaches and make your fasting days miserable and harder. So unless you have other reasons to give up caffeine just work out your normal consumption and make sure you count all the calories you have in your caffeinated drinks.

There are lots of ways to get your normal caffeine hit without adding any calories. Black tea and coffee and diet sodas/energy drinks are the obvious choice. The calories in these drinks are insignificant.

But if your preferred drink is tea or coffee with milk or cream then don't cut it out. Just make sure you count the calories in each cup. You should also consider switching to skim milk which has 40 cals per ½ cup as opposed to 2% which has 61 cals per ½ cup.

Finally, I must admit that my breakfast choice from the above list is ALWAYS a skinny latte. I make my own and have perfected the recipe over the years. I have included it in the recipes section of the book. For reference a short (8oz) skinny latte from Starbucks is 70 cals and a tall (12oz) skinny latte is 100 cals. Other coffee outlets are similar.

Q: Should I exercise as normal?

A: Not on your diet days

When you start the 5:2 diet you may be wondering what to do about your normal exercise routine. In the first few weeks at least you should not try and exercise on your diet days. This is for two reasons. Firstly, you may feel physically weaker on your fasting days when you start this diet – this wears off soon. Secondly, exercising will simply make you more hungry – something you want to avoid at this stage. You do however have 5 non-diet days for whatever exercise routine you normally do (or don't!) follow.

Q: What about alcoholic beverages?

A: Not on your diet days

Alcoholic beverages contain plenty of calories and will probably make you feel light-headed on your diet days so it's worth steering clear of alcoholic drinks on these days. Of course you're free to do what you want on the other 5 days.

Q: What should I eat on a feast (non-diet) day?

A: Whatever you like

The first rule for feast days is there are no rules! You can eat what you want and really enjoy it. This is your reward for the fast day before. Your body will regulate itself and even on the day after a fast day you'll at most eat 10% - 15% more than normal.

Be aware that on the first day after a fast day the breakfast that you've been looking forward to may be a bit of a let down. You'll be surprised that you cannot manage to eat as much as you thought you wanted. You may also feel rather tired and lethargic that first feast day. This is just your body compensating for the fast day. As your body gets used to fasting this won't happen and feast days will be trouble-free.

Week-by-week guide

Week One

You've chosen your diet days and your menu plan. You've read up on what you can and cannot eat. You're ready and raring to go. So let's get started.

Week 1, day 1 is probably going to be your hardest. It is the day when you have to be strictest about counting calories and the day you are likely to feel the hungriest. Yet it is also the day when you are most motivated. Think positively and just remember you only have to experience it once and you will find day 2 much easier. Just think of the all the lovely food you can eat tomorrow and maybe check if your stomach is just a little bit flatter.

You may also be able to get on the scales the morning after your first fasting day and see a drop of a pound or two. How's that for motivation?

In your first week, you should be very aware of what you are eating and when you eat.

Make the most of the calories you can eat and eat things that will fill you up for longer with the least amount of calories. This generally means eating mainly proteins – eggs, chicken or fish – with plenty of vegetables and salad. Carbohydrates like bread, pasta and rice contain lots of calories and you will burn up the energy and be hungry again quickly afterwards.

Beware of what you drink. There are plenty of no calorie or low calorie drinks out there. Water, diet sodas, black tea or coffee are all fine. But drinks with milk add calories and a simple glass of orange juice could have nearly 100 calories.

Check the labels on everything you eat. Most food bought from supermarkets now has an exact calorie count for each item. This will be more accurate than the necessarily more general advice given here. Get your calculator out and add in every little thing.

The easiest way to follow the 5:2 diet in the first week is to stick to a menu plan. Remember that you can adapt the examples given here if you find it easier to eat at different times or if you've got different things in your cupboard.

Take it easy and even try and enjoy it. Relish your non-diet days and congratulate yourself at the end of each diet day.

Benefits you are likely to see in the first week

If you've made it through the first two days of fasting then you should be congratulating yourself. The next week's fasting days will be so much easier. Benefits such as increased energy are coming soon. But the thing you'll notice first will be weight-loss. You will be at your lightest before you eat at the start of the day following the second fast day. How much you lose will be determined by your starting weight and your body type. But some weight-loss is pretty much guaranteed.

Week Two

In Week 2 you should follow an almost identical pattern to week 1 but you will find it significantly easier.

Week 2 is all about building on week 1 and getting your body used to fasting. You should find the hunger pangs are less frequent and milder.

Weeks Three and Four

In weeks 3 and 4 your diet days are no longer a shock to the system. As your body is now used to the diet it should be getting significantly easier. You are unlikely to feel light-headed or grumpy during the day as your body is now finding the diet more natural.

In fact, the human body is not particularly designed for a regular daily calorie intake; this is a more modern invention. Back in the days of hunter-gatherers good meals were infrequent and they necessarily only ate by feast and famine. Our bodies are still built to cope well with this and the 5:2 diet is just trying to adapt the body back to this state.

If you've been following one of the menu plans then you finish your plan at the end of week 3. There's nothing to stop you starting again at the beginning in week 4, but now is the time that you'll probably want to adapt the diet a little to suit your needs. You'll be feeling more comfortable about how the 5:2 works and have found some recipes that you like and that fit your lifestyle. If there's any particular aspect of the menu plan you found hard it's worth trying out one of the other plans and seeing if it suits you better.

Mainly you should still consider the menu plan your guide; feel free to branch out, try some other recipes and generally make the 5:2 diet your own.

Benefits you are likely to see in the first month

As you near the end of your first month of 5:2 dieting you will find that your body has adapted fully to this diet as a way of life. I hope that you can begin to enjoy your fasting days and to feel healthier in body and spirit.

As well as continuing to lose weight (and doesn't that feel good!) you may well notice an increase in energy. Contrary to what you might expect on a diet day you feel energized and ready for anything.

Also, under the hood and hard to measure, the longer-term health benefits should be starting to kick in. If you started with raised cholesterol levels they may have started to drop. And even though you might not be able to see them outwardly some of those longer term, age-related health risks will now be reducing.

Into the future

If you've made it this far then all you need to do is carry on in exactly the same way and continue to reap the benefits. The 5:2 diet is not a fad; you should find it easy to carry it on for years to come. More than that you should want to keep doing it because it's so simple to follow and the benefits are so amazing.

By all means take a break for Christmas or when you go on holiday, you deserve it. And you know that you can just kick back into the diet when you get back and those holiday pounds will soon disappear.

I hope that above all you can see the 5:2 diet positively as something that you can continue. To many people who start down this route it is not a diet; it is a way of life that allows them to maintain a healthy weight while eating what they want. And according to research they are gaining great long term health benefits too.

Extending your weight-loss

If you have found that your weight-loss has slowed down and you feel like you need a little extra diet boost you could consider an occasional extra diet day or adding in gentle exercise on a diet day.

Low intensity exercise

Add half an hour of low intensity exercise such as walking, swimming or a light gym session on your fasting days.

Choose whatever exercise suits you best; it can be as simple as a gentle walk. You can fit the exercise in whenever you like during the day. A particularly nice time to exercise is in the evening as you will have less time to feel hungry afterwards and it's often a nice way to end the day. The most important thing to remember is not to push yourself as you won't have as much strength as on a normal day. Note that you can carry on exercising as normal (or not) on your feast days.

Exercise adds the following advantages to your 5:2 diet:

- improves your body shape and tone more than exercising on your feast days
- increases your weight-loss
- gives you more vitality
- distraction from hunger pangs
- exercise is less punishing and more fun

Occasional third diet day

If the 5:2 fasting is continuing to work well for you then this option is not for you. You should only consider fasting an extra day if you have been successfully following the 5:2 diet for at least six weeks and are finding that your body has fully adjusted to fasting days. This does not add to the health benefits of fasting but can give your weight-loss a boost.

Adding a third fast day in a week could be considered when one or more of the following are true:

- you have reached a weight-loss plateau
- you are preparing for a party or event and want to look your best the next day
- as a pre-emptive measure – you have a big party or event ahead of you and you want to be able to eat and drink more than normal without the usual guilt

The rules for a third day of fasting are effectively the same as for the other fasting days. You must have a feast day between each fast day.

I would not advise this as a normal course of events. I would advise it only occasionally, say once a month at most to have the most effect.

Personally I find a third fast day rather hard to fit into my normal routine and only do it very rarely. What I have found works well for me instead is an extra half day.

2 ½ fast days and 4 ½ feast days

It's not exactly a good name for a diet is it? This is something I follow more often than not as it fits practically into my life. Let me explain.

When I am thinking about which days to fast each week I normally reach the following conclusion:

I don't want to fast at the weekend. Therefore, Monday is an obvious fast day. I know this is the choice of the majority of 5:2 dieters. Tuesday must then be a feast day which leaves Wednesday or Thursday for fasting. If Wednesday fits suitably into my calendar I tend to go for Wednesday. Which means if I want to add an extra fast day into my week then it would need to be on Friday. BUT I have a problem with Fridays. On Fridays I might want to go out in the evening and if not I'll be most likely wanting a relaxing glass of wine at home to celebrate the start of the weekend.

I think more than one of you reading this must have reached a similar conclusion. So I have found a third option for ultimate weight-loss that does not rule out any of my normal treats.

Monday: fast day, 500 (650 for men) calories

Tuesday: feast day

Wednesday: fast day, 500 (650 for men) calories

Thursday: feast day

Friday: **fast day until 6pm**

On Friday (or whichever day you choose for a half-day fast) you should follow normal fasting rules until 6pm and then anything goes. So you would have your standard meagre breakfast on Friday and then fast until 6pm. But at 6pm you can eat normally and no longer count calories. This works because the fast is long enough to shake your body into fasting mode. Also, it is hard to eat a full day's worth of calories in the evening. I estimate that even with pizza, wine and cookies (a typical Friday evening in our house!) my calorie count for the half day is about 1000 calories. But I don't calorie count on the Friday; I just enjoy my evening as well-earned and am all set for a relaxing and fun weekend.

Maintaining your weight

What if you've been following the 5:2 diet for a while and you are now at your target weight? Do you want to continue to have the health benefits of the 5:2 diet but you don't want to actually lose any more weight?

The simple answer is to cut back your fasting days to one a week. This is maintenance mode and you shouldn't lose weight with only fasting one day a week. If you continue to lose weight you could always stop altogether for a month or so and then do occasional fasting days.

We don't know whether one day a week of calorie restriction is enough to get all the health benefits, but in as much as we do know today it is likely that you will continue to cut your risk factors for age-related diseases.

How the 5:2 diet can help you live longer

So what about the amazing health benefits of which we've seen such tantalizing glimpses? A healthy long-life and a lower risk of heart disease, cancer and Alzheimer's. If this is all true then surely everyone would be on this diet?

Until very recently fasting was considered one of the more extreme dieting options; shunned by the mainstream medical profession as dangerous. It is only with this new breed of short non-total fasts, of which the 5:2 diet is the most popular and the easiest, that intermittent fasting is becoming more recognized as an option.

As a result research into short-term fasting is still in its infancy. At present we have a small selection of interesting studies from both sides of the Atlantic which have all produced some encouraging results. We have Professor Longo in California, who has been investigating the effects of the growth hormone IGF-1; research at Manchester University into the reduction of cancer risks; studies at Newcastle University into reversal of Type 2 diabetes through fasting; Krista Varady's research in Chicago into reducing the risk factors of heart disease; and research in Baltimore into how the 5:2 diet may protect us against brain diseases such as Alzheimer's.

We should do well to remember that as yet there are no long-term studies into the results of intermittent fasting; for this we have to look into the past and learn from history and some of the great world religions.

Professor Valter Longo at the Longevity Institute at the University of Southern California has been investigating insulin-like growth factor 1 (known as IGF-1), a hormone produced in the liver which keeps our cells growing.

When we eat normally our cells are constantly active and grow too fast for damage to be repaired effectively. When we fast levels of IGF-1 drop and we enter a state known as "autophagy" where our bodies produce fewer new cells and concentrate on repairing old ones. This effectively slows the aging process while we fast.

Professor Longo has been working with Laron mice, which have been genetically engineered so that they don't respond to IGF-1. These mice are very small and exceptionally long-lived. They can live for up to five years which is more than twice the expected life-span of a normal mouse. In human terms that's equivalent to living to as much as 160 years old. Additionally these mice are pretty much immune to heart disease and cancer, and simply die of old age when their time comes.

Longo has also studied villagers from a remote community in Ecuador who have a genetic defect known as Laron syndrome. This is incredibly rare, affecting less than 350 people world-wide. People with Laron syndrome are short (less than 4ft tall) and, like the Laron mice, do not respond to IGF-1. They are also long-lived (although not exceptionally so). Most interestingly of all they appear to be resistant to cancer, diabetes and heart disease; there is not a single known case of someone with Laron syndrome dying of cancer.

The research by Professor Longo has shown that fasting lowers levels of IGF-1 and switches on DNA repair genes. Simply put, when our bodies run out of food our cells change from "growth" to "repair" mode.

Another study, this time from the National Institute on Ageing in Baltimore, has shown that reducing your calorie intake two days a week (i.e. the 5:2 diet) may protect against Alzheimer's, Parkinson's and other degenerative brain conditions. Professor

Mark Mattson, who has led the study at the institute's laboratory of neurosciences, says that he and his colleagues have worked out a mechanism by which the growth of neurones in the brain could be affected by reduced calorie intakes. Intermittent fasting increases nerve cell growth factor which in turn protects neurons in the brain against the adversities of ageing. This may well reduce the risk factors for cognitive diseases such as Alzheimer's.

Mattson insists there are evolutionary reasons for believing it to be the case. "When resources became scarce, our ancestors would have had to scrounge for food," said Mattson. "Those whose brains responded best – who remembered where promising sources of food could be found or recalled how to avoid predators – would have been the ones who got the food. Thus a mechanism linking periods of starvation to neural growth would have evolved."

As we have seen in other studies this research is still in it's early stages, with human studies only just beginning.

In the UK a study by researchers at Newcastle University into the effects of fasting on sufferers of Type 2 diabetes has had some incredible results. In an early stage clinical trial all 11 volunteers reversed their diabetes by drastically cutting their food intake to just 600 calories a day for two months. And three months after the diet finished 70% remained free of diabetes. Professor Roy Taylor of Newcastle University who led the study said: "To have people free of diabetes after years with the condition is remarkable – and all because of an eight week diet."

Participants on the study found the diet very, very difficult to stick to and were only able to do so with the close supervision of a medical team. But for these volunteers the results were astonishing. Most were taking diabetes medicine before the trial and at the end found their insulin levels to be normal and that they no longer needed their medication.

Also in the UK, this time at the University of Manchester, a study of women following a strict 650 calorie diet just two days a week were found to lower their risk of breast cancer by 40%. The study, led by Dr Michelle Harvie, examined 50 overweight women from Greater Manchester. After six months following a 650-calorie-a-day diet for two days a week (and eating normally the rest of the week) the women had dropped an average of 13lb and showed major improvements in key areas linked to breast cancer. The women found their levels of the hormone leptin (known as a cancer risk factor) dropped 40% and their insulin levels dropped by up to 25%. Pamela Goldberg, chief executive of the Breast Cancer Campaign, said "This intermittent dieting approach provides an alternative to conventional dieting which could help with weight loss, but also potentially reduce the risk of developing breast cancer."

Finally, and perhaps the most relevant study, is on-going research by Dr Krista Varady at the University of Illinois at Chicago. Dr Varady has been studying a diet known as ADF, Alternate Day Fasting, where you eat restricted calories (600 for a man, 500 for a woman) every other day. The 5:2 diet is a less dramatic variant of the same diet. Dr Varady's research has three main aims: to find a diet that people can stick to for long periods of time, to see what weight-loss can be expected when following ADF for up to a year and to study the effect of intermittent fasting on certain heart disease risk factors, such as cholesterol and blood pressure.

As the study is still progressing the final conclusion is unavailable. Initial results are promising, however, with a low drop-out rate, gradual and continued weight-loss in most subjects and some impressive falls in cholesterol (down 21%), LDL ("bad") cholesterol (down 25%) and blood pressure.

Another interesting trial from Dr Varady took two groups of volunteers doing ADF for 10 weeks. One group were put on a low-fat diet on their feast days, while the other were encouraged to eat a typical high-fat American diet. Everyone, including Dr Varady, expected that the high-fat group would lose less weight than those following the low-fat diet. But they didn't, people on the high-fat diet were losing as much and sometimes even more weight, week after week. This suggests that we can eat what we want on our non-diet days as it really makes no difference.

The recipes

This is a book of ideas for eating healthy, well-balanced and low calorie food, perfect for the days when you have to watch your calories.

Every recipe here is specifically designed to keep you feeling satisfied for longer. This is done by choosing lean proteins, low fats and complex carbohydrates and combining them with bold flavors. Although a few recipes require a smaller portion size most provide you with a healthy "normal" plate of food.

The majority of recipes are for one portion but could be doubled up. Where this isn't practical the recipe makes two servings, suitable for sharing with your partner or keeping for another day. There are also plenty of recipes that are suitable to serve to your family.

The recipes include some practical suggestions for making larger quantities for freezing so you have a selection of frozen meals to choose from. You can then take a portion to work or have one ready when you get home with a minimal amount of fuss.

Finally, everything is simple to prepare and cook. The ingredients are all readily available in any grocery store. There's nothing too fancy or expensive here.

So please use this as an inspiration and a starting point for your own 5:2 cooking. Just because you're on a diet (for 1 day!) doesn't mean you have to be hungry...

Breakfast ideas

Under 100 calories

A perfect Caffé Latte at home
40 calories per cup

Serves 1 Cook time: 3m

½ cup skim milk
½ cup good-quality brewed coffee
OR
1 generous scoop or tablespoon of good quality ground coffee
½ cup boiling water
French Press or other coffee brewing device

If using a French Press, pour ½ cup boiling water over your coffee. Leave to brew for 2 minutes. Meanwhile heat ½ cup skim milk until it is warm. Too hot and it will form a skin. You can do this on the stovetop until the milk gives off the first hint of steam or by giving it approximately 40 seconds in the microwave on high. When the coffee has brewed for two minutes plunge the French Press (or measure out ½ cup from your coffee maker) and pour into the warm milk. If using a French Press, make sure you get the last dregs of the coffee as this gives it its froth. Now get the coffee back up to temp by giving it another microwave blast of about 30 seconds.

Blackberry fool
45 calories per serving

Serves 1 Prep time: 2m

¼ cup blackberries
¼ cup fat-free Greek yogurt
1 tsp calorie-free sweetener

Mash the blackberries slightly with a fork and fold in the Greek yogurt.

Egg white omelet
57 calories per serving

Serves 1 Prep time: 2m Cook time: 2m

3 large eggs
3 sprays of olive oil cooking spray, like Pam Organic Olive Oil Spray

First separate your eggs. Have 2 bowls in front of you. Crack the egg on the side of one of the bowls. Holding the egg over one of the bowls, carefully transfer the egg yolk back and forth from one half of the shell to the other, letting the egg white drip out into the bowl below. Keep transferring the yolk back and forth until all the white is in the bowl. Then put the yolk in the second bowl. Repeat for the other 2 eggs. Whisk the egg whites together using a fork.

Spray your oil into a wide non-stick skillet and pre-heat at a medium setting for at least 2 minutes. Then add your egg whites. Sprinkle on plenty of salt and pepper. The omelet should cook in less than a minute. Serve immediately.

Yogurt with blueberries
86 calories per serving

Serves 1 Prep time: 2m

½ cup low fat plain yogurt
⅓ cup blueberries
1 tsp calorie-free sweetener

Place blueberries in a bowl and mash lightly with a fork. Stir in the yogurt.

Hot chocolate
102 calories per serving

Serves 1 Cook time: 2m

1 cup skim milk
1 tsp cocoa
1 tsp sugar

Heat the milk gently on the hob until lightly steaming or in the microwave for approximately one minute. Stir in the cocoa and sugar.

Under 150 calories

Oatmeal pot
150 calories per serving

Oatmeal is a tasty, warming and filling breakfast. This is an Oatmeal pot because it's about half of a normal serving. Serve in a small dish such as a ramekin.

Serves 1 Cook time: 3m

¼ cup rolled porridge oats
¾ cup skim milk

In a large bowl or glass measuring cup stir the milk into the oats. Heat in the microwave on high for two minutes. Consistency is everything with porridge; it should be thick without being gelatinous and liquid without being runny. If it's too thick add in some more milk a little at a time while stirring. If it's too thin, stir and microwave for another 30 seconds.

Under 200 calories

"Fast" food breakfast sandwich
197 calories per serving

Faster than driving through your local fast food breakfast place – and at less than 200 calories, leaves you plenty of calories to work with for the rest of your fast day.

Serves 1 Cook time: 8m

1 Pepperidge Farm "Deli Flat" sandwich roll
2 sprays of olive oil cooking spray
1 slice Oscar Mayer Canadian Bacon
1 large egg

Pop your Deli Flat roll in the toaster, and spray a non-stick skillet with the olive oil spray. Cook your egg and Canadian bacon slice in the skillet over medium heat until the bacon is a bit brown and the egg is cooked as you like it. I like the yolk runny if I'm eating at home, but if you're on the go, you'll probably want to cook it hard!.You can use a silicon egg ring if you want to keep your egg perfectly round and neat.

Bacon, eggs, and toast
184 calories per serving

Serves 1 Cook time: 10m

2 slices of turkey bacon
1 large egg
1 slice Pepperidge Farm Very Thin bread
3 sprays olive oil cooking spray

Heat a large non-stick skillet over medium heat for 2 minutes before adding the ingredients. Spray the oil into the pan to prevent sticking. Fry the bacon for about 3 minutes or until it's almost as done as you like. Pop the bread into the toaster, then turn the bacon and add the egg into the pan as well. Your egg should finish cooking just about the time your toast pops up!

Breakfast Burrito
185 calories per serving

Serves 1 Cook time: 10m

1 low-calorie tortilla
2 egg whites lightly beaten with salt and pepper (see page 38 for easy instructions on separating eggs)
½ bell pepper
½ small onion
3 thin slices of healthy deli turkey or ham
4 sprays of olive oil cooking spray
2 tbsp salsa
2 tbsp plain, fat-free yogurt

Dice the pepper, onions, and turkey/ham, and cook over medium-low heat in a skillet with the cooking spray. Once the onions go a bit translucent, add the beaten egg whites and scramble just until set. Heat tortilla for 10 seconds on a plate in the microwave. Fill with the scrambled egg whites and top with the salsa and yogurt, tuck in the ends, and roll up!

Home-made granola
199 calories per serving (inc. ½ cup skim milk)

Serves 8 Prep time: 10m Cook time: 15m

1½ cups rolled oats
1 tbsp pumpkin seeds
1 tbsp sunflower seeds
¼ cup pistachios, shelled and chopped
¼ cup almonds, chopped
juice of 1 lemon
1 tbsp honey
¼ cup raisins

Mix the oats, seeds and nuts together in a bowl. Stir together the lemon juice and honey and add to the dry ingredients, mixing well.

Spread evenly over a large baking sheet and bake in a pre-heated oven at 350F for 10 minutes. Add the raisins to the baking sheet and bake for a another 5 minutes. When cool can be stored in an airtight container for up to 2 weeks. Serve with ½ cup of skim milk.

Under 300 calories

Scrambled eggs with peppers and tomatoes
249 calories per serving

Originally from the Basque region of France, this is scrambled eggs like you've never seen them before.

Serves 1 Prep time: 5m Cook time: 15m

1 tsp olive oil
½ onion, finely diced
1 clove garlic, sliced
1 red pepper, de-seeded and diced
½ 14oz can can of diced tomatoes
1 large egg
1 egg white (see egg white omelet on page 38 for instructions on how to separate an egg)
3 fresh basil leaves if you have them

Heat the oil in a frying pan and add the onions, garlic and peppers. Sauté them gently on a medium heat for 8 minutes, until golden. Add the diced tomatoes and cook for another 5 minutes.

Meanwhile, whisk together the egg and egg white and season with salt and pepper. Pour the eggs into the frying pan with the other ingredients, stirring constantly until they thicken like scrambled eggs – about 3 minutes. Serve with basil on the top.

Salads

Under 100 calories

Standard salad
78 calories per serving (including salad dressing)

A lot of the recipes listed later on call for a salad as an accompaniment. Here is what I would put into a standard salad for one person, totalling 68 calories per portion.

Serves 1 Prep time: 5m

¼ iceberg lettuce
2 inches cucumber
2 medium (2 inch diameter) tomatoes

Using 1 tablespoon of pre-bought light salad dressing will add 10 calories.

"German" salad
94 calories per serving (including dressing)

Add a little variety to your salads...

Serves 1 Prep time: 5m

¼ iceberg lettuce
2 inches cucumber
2 medium (2 inch diameter) tomatoes
1 large or 3 small sweet pickles
2 tsp capers
1 tbsp extra-light Miracle Whip or Mayonnaise

Ham or bacon salad
98 calories per serving

A little bit more filling than a standard salad.

¼ iceberg lettuce
2 inches cucumber
1 medium (2 inch diameter) tomato
1 slice of ham, diced, or 1 slice turkey bacon, cooked and crumbled
1 tbsp light salad dressing

Under 200 calories

Chargrilled vegetable salad
127 calories per serving

You prepare this salad by cooking the vegetables in a grill pan or heavy frying pan and then marinating overnight – or you could cut into chunks instead of slices, put them on skewers and cook on the grill, if you happen to be using it the day before a fast day. Ideal for preparing the night before and taking to work the next day.

Serves 2 Prep time: 10m Cook time: 10m Marinate time: 8h

4 sprays olive oil cooking spray
1 small eggplant sliced across the width into thin slices
1 zucchini sliced lengthways thinly
4 spring onions
1 red pepper, de-seeded and quartered
6 asparagus spears

½ shallot, diced
½ red chili, de-seeded and finely sliced
1 clove garlic, sliced

4 basil leaves, shredded
1 tbsp extra virgin olive oil
2 tsp red wine vinegar

Use a grill pan if you've got one – if not, a normal frying pan will do fine. Spray the pan with the 4 sprays of oil and heat to medium-high. Cook all the vegetables for about 10 minutes, turning once, until browned on the edges. You may need to do this in two separate batches. If cooking the vegetables on skewers on the grill, remember to spray the vegetables with the cooking spray, not the grill – the fire could flash back and be really dangerous!

Combine the diced shallot, chili, garlic, basil, oil and vinegar in a dish and toss over the vegetables while they are still warm. Make sure all the vegetables are covered in the marinade before leaving overnight to marinate. Serve at room temperature.

Oriental shrimp and mushroom salad
151 calories per serving

Serves 1 Prep time: 5m

1 cup mushrooms, washed and finely sliced
3oz jumbo shrimp, cooked
2 cups baby spinach or other salad leaves
1 spring onion, sliced
2 tsp rice vinegar
juice ½ lemon
1 tsp light soy sauce
1 tsp olive oil

Cut the shrimp in half and combine with the mushrooms, spring onion and salad leaves. In a small bowl mix together the rice vinegar, lemon juice, soy sauce and olive oil. Pour the dressing over the salad and toss well.

Italian bread salad
170 calories per serving

Serves 1 Prep time: 5m Marinate time: 30m

½ thick slice whole grain bread
6 ripe cherry tomatoes, quartered
1 spring onion, sliced
2 inches cucumber, diced
½ clove garlic, crushed
2 basil leaves, shredded
1 tsp extra virgin olive oil
2 tsp red wine vinegar

This salad is best if the bread is slightly stale. Remove the crust from the bread and cut into chunks. Place the bread in a bowl and sprinkle with a little water. Add the tomatoes, spring onion, cucumber and celery and mix gently. In a small bowl mix together the garlic, basil, olive oil and red wine vinegar to make the dressing and pour over the salad. Leave for half an hour at room temperature for the flavors to develop.

Warm bean salad
199 calories per serving

Serves 1 Prep time: 2m Cook time: 4m

¼ 14oz can of mixed beans
½ cup green beans, fresh or frozen
2 tsp extra virgin olive oil
juice of ½ lemon
salt and pepper

Place the mixed beans in a small saucepan and add just enough water to cover them. Warm through on a medium heat for 5 minutes. Meanwhile boil your green beans for 3 minutes. Drain both your mixed beans and your green beans and place in a bowl. While still warm mix in the oil, lemon juice and seasoning.

Under 300 calories

Shrimp, wild rice and arugula salad
211 calories per serving

Serves 1 Cook time: 30m Prep time: 2m

¼ cup red or wild rice
3oz shrimp, cooked (if frozen, defrosted)
2 cups of arugula (or baby spinach)
juice of ½ lemon
½ tsp extra virgin olive oil
freshly ground black pepper

Cook the rice in boiling water for 30 minutes, or as per pack instructions if different. Drain and leave to cool. In a bowl mix together the rice and rocket and then place the shrimp on the top. Squeeze over the lemon juice and a small drizzle (½ teaspoon) of olive oil. Finally sprinkle on a little black pepper.

Salade Nicoise
292 calories per serving

A classic; substantial and tasty.

Serves 1 Prep time: 10m

1 head of Boston or butter lettuce separated into leaves
1 tomato, quartered
1 hard-boiled egg, cut into quarters
½ cup green beans, cooked (from fresh or frozen)
½ 6oz can of tuna in water or brine
1 anchovy fillet, dried on kitchen paper
5 black olives

For the dressing:
1 tsp extra virgin olive oil
1 tsp white wine vinegar
1 tsp capers
salt and pepper

Mix together the dressing ingredients and set aside. Place the lettuce leaves in a bowl and add the tomato, green beans and hard-boiled egg. Roughly flake the tuna and add in. Pour the dressing over the salad. Top with the anchovy fillet and scatter over the olives.

Egyptian chicken salad
293 calories per serving

Serves 2 Prep time: 10m

2 chicken breasts, cooked (approx 12oz)
3 inches cucumber, roughly cubed
10 cherry tomatoes, halved
½ red pepper, diced
2 spring onions, finely chopped
4 mint leaves, shredded
4 parsley leaves, shredded
2 Romaine hearts, chopped
For the dressing:
2 tsp extra virgin olive oil
juice of 1 lemon
½ clove garlic, finely chopped
1 tsp ground cumin
salt and pepper

Mix together the dressing ingredients in a small cup or bowl and set aside to rest for 5 minutes. Place the chicken, cucumber, tomatoes, red pepper, spring onions, lettuce and herbs in another large bowl and toss the dressing over, making sure everything is well coated.

Warm leek and lentil salad with goat's cheese
298 calories per serving

This is an extremely filling and warming dish.

Serves 1 Prep time: 5m Soak time: 15m Cook time: 30m

¼ cup puy lentils (dry weight)
2 leeks
2 sprays olive oil cooking spray
½ clove garlic, finely chopped
5 sun-dried tomatoes
1oz light feta/Greek style cheese
few drops balsamic vinegar

Put the dried tomatoes in a small cup. Pour in boiling water so the cup is about ¼ full. Leave to soak. Wash the lentils under running water for a minute before transferring to a small saucepan and covering with about an inch of cold water. Bring up to the boil and simmer gently for 25 minutes until cooked. Top up with more water if it starts to look dry.

Meanwhile chop your leeks finely. In a wide saucepan with a lid, add a few sprays of light oil and when at a medium heat add the leeks and garlic and fry for 3-4 minutes. As the leeks start to brown add half a cup of water, stir and put the lid on the pan. Cook for another 6 minutes. Chop the feta into very small squares. Remove the tomatoes from their soaking liquid and cut into small pieces. Stir the tomatoes and lentils into the leeks. Place in a bowl and top with the feta and a drizzle of balsamic vinegar.

Light lunches

As you may well have already found the nation's lunch-time staple, bread (in all its many forms), contains a substantial number of calories. Most of the lunch choices in this section contain bread, pita or flatbread because that is what we enjoy and find convenient for our lunch-time meal. However, we need to make clever choices to ensure the meal does not contain too many calories. To do this it is easiest to buy reduced calorie bread products which have clear labeling on the number of calories per slice. I only use bread products that you can buy from any grocery Here are some of the best that I have found:

Pepperidge Farm Deli Flats, Bagel Flats, and Very Thin Bread

The flats are small rolls or buns that come pre-sliced, ready to toast or fill as you like – at 100 calories each. The Very Thin Bread is exactly as described – normal bread, sliced thinner than you'd think was possible, at 50 calories per slice for white, 60 calories per slice for wheat.

Crispbreads (like RyKrisp) – (around 30 calories each but check package)

Rice Cakes (30 calories)

Low calorie tortillas (80 calories)

Pita bread (60-90 calories per half pita, check label)

Under 150 calories

Crispbread with peanut butter and tomato
88 calories per serving

This is a favorite snack of mine. My husband thinks I'm weird, but I find the tomato takes off the sometimes cloying edge of the peanut butter and the balsamic gives it an extra zing.

Serves 1 Preparation time: 2m

1 slice crispbread
2 tsp natural (unsweetened) peanut butter
1 slice tomato
few drops of balsamic vinegar

Spread the peanut butter evenly over the crispbread and top with the slice of tomato. Drizzle a little balsamic over the top.

Pastrami on RyKrisp
120 calories per serving

Serves 1 Preparation time: 5m

2 slices RyKrisp Crispbread
2 tsp mustard
4 slices pastrami
2 small sweet pickles, sliced

Spread the mustard thinly over the RyKrisp. Place two slices of pastrami on each. Slice the pickles extremely thinly lengthways and lay evenly over the pastrami.

Crispbread with cream cheese and cucumber
140 calories per serving

Serves 1 Prep time: 2m

1 slice crispbread
2 tablespoon slight cream cheese
4 thick slices cucumber

Spread an even quantity of cream cheese on each crispbread and top with two slices of cucumber each. Season with salt and pepper.

Home-made salsa on flatbread
144 calories per serving

This works great with Pepperidge Farm Deli Flats, but any diet bread that equals 100 calories per serving would be great in this recipe.

Salsa serves 4 Prep time: 10m Infuse time: 1h

¼ red onion
1 green chili, de-seeded
1 spring onion
1 clove garlic
4 tomatoes
1 tsp olive oil
½ to 1 tsp salt
juice of 1 lemon
1 tsp tomato purée
1 tbsp water
1 flatbread

Combine the red onion, green chili, spring onion and garlic in a food processor. Whizz until finely chopped. Add the tomatoes (whole, with skins and seeds all ok!), olive oil, salt, lemon juice, tomato purée and water. Pulse the food processor until just chopped; you want it chunky. Transfer to a bowl and check the salt. Leave for ½ to 1 hour for the flavours to infuse.

Serve by spreading ¼ of the mix generously over a toasted flatbread.

Under 200 calories

Smoked salmon and cream cheese on crispbread
169 calories per serving

Serves 1 Prep time: 5m

4 slices of crispbread
4 tsp low-fat cream cheese
1 slice smoked salmon (¾oz)
1 slice lemon
freshly ground black pepper

Spread 1 teaspoon of cream cheese on each crispbread and top with ¼ of the salmon. Top each with ¼ of the remaining cream cheese. Squeeze on a little lemon juice and add a sprinkling of black pepper.

Cucumber dip with home-made tortilla chips
180 calories per serving

Serves 2 Prep time: 5m Infuse time: 30m Cook time: 5m

1 cup plain, fat-free yogurt
2 inches cucumber
2 tsp dried mint
pinch of salt
1 tsp extra virgin olive oil
2 low calorie tortillas

Peel and coarsely grate the cucumber. Place in a small bowl with the yogurt, mint and a pinch of salt. Stir well and leave for 30 minutes at room temperature for the flavors to develop.

Cut your tortillas into small triangles and place on a non-stick baking tray. Pre-heat the oven to 450F and cook the tortilla chips for 4-5 minutes until golden brown. Remove from the oven and allow to cool on the baking sheet for a few minutes until they're crispy.

Place the dip in a serving dish and drizzle with the olive oil. Serve the tortilla chips on a plate surrounding the dip.

Open-faced BLT
186 calories per serving

You won't feel like you're dieting if you have one of these!

Prep time: 2m Cook time: 5m

1 slice Pepperidge Farm Very Thin Bread, or half of a Pepperidge Farm Deli Flat (50 cal total)
3 slices turkey bacon
1 tbsp light mayonnaise
2 slices of tomato
finely sliced lettuce

Cook the bacon in a dry, non-stick skillet. Lightly toast the flatbread. Spread the mayonnaise thinly over the flatbread and top with the lettuce. Put the bacon on next and finally add the sliced tomato.

Easy hummus with vegetables for dipping
195 calories per serving

Makes 8 servings of hummus (139 calories per serving)

Prep time: 10m

1 14oz can chick peas
5 tbsp tahini paste
2 cloves garlic, peeled
juice of 2 lemons
2 tbsp olive oil
pinch cayenne pepper
salt and pepper

For dipping, per person:
½ red pepper, de-seeded and sliced into sticks
2 inches cucumber, cut into sticks
½ carrot, peeled and cut into sticks

Blitz the chick peas and garlic in a food processor with a little water from the can until smooth. Add the tahini, lemon juice, cayenne pepper and a good pinch of salt and pepper. Blitz again until really smooth. Turn into a dish or individual portions. Can keep for up to 3 days in the fridge. Serve an individual portion in a small dish or ramekin, surrounded by the vegetable sticks.

Ham omelet
198 calories per serving

You probably don't need instructions for this, but I've included them just in case.

Serves 1 Prep time: 2m Cook time:3m

2 large eggs
2 slices of healthy, deli-style ham, cut into pieces
4 sprays of olive oil cooking spray

Put the eggs and a tablespoon of water in a bowl. Whisk the eggs together using a fork. Pour them into a hot, oiled frying pan, making sure they cover the bottom. After about 30 seconds lift up one side of the omelet with a wooden spoon and tilt the pan slightly to allow some of the uncooked egg to fill the gap. Repeat all around the omelet until it no longer runs. Spread the ham evenly over the top. Give it another 30 seconds before folding and sliding onto a plate.

Under 300 calories

Refried beans and goat's cheese hot wrap
228 calories per serving

Serves 1 Prep time: 5m Cook time: 5m

1 low-calorie tortilla
¼ 14oz can of kidney or light red beans
few sprays olive oil cooking spray
few drops Worcestershire sauce
¾oz light goat's cheese
1 tomato
1 inch cucumber
juice of ½ lime

Put the kidney beans into a colander and rinse. Using a fork gently press on the beans so they are broken up but not mashed.

Heat a small saucepan with the oil spray and add the kidney beans. Add salt and pepper and a few drops of Worcestershire sauce. Fry for about 5 minutes stirring occasionally until the beans start to go brown and crunchy.

Meanwhile prepare the goat's cheese salad. Chop the goat's cheese into very small cubes and place in a bowl. Cut the tomato and cucumber into small cubes and add to the bowl. Squeeze over the juice of the lime and stir in.

Heat the tortilla in the microwave for 10 seconds. Lay it flat on a plate and spread the beans over the top, leaving an inch free at the bottom to fold over. Arrange the goat's cheese salad over the beans. Fold up the bottom inch and then roll up the wrap.

Watercress falafel
230 calories per serving

Serve on a bed of watercress with lemon wedges on the side.

Serves 2 Prep time: 5m Cook time: 20m

1 14oz can chickpeas, rinsed and drained
¼ cup watercress
1 tablespoon tahini paste
1 clove garlic, peeled
juice ½ lemon
1 tsp baking powder
1 tsp cumin
½ tsp cayenne pepper
2 tsp olive oil

Place all the ingredients except the oil in a food processor and whizz until finely chopped but not puréed. Shape the mixture into 6 balls and flatten slightly with the palm of your hand. Brush the falafel with a little olive oil on both sides and arrange on a non-stick baking tray. Cook in a pre-heated oven at 400F for 18-20 minutes until golden brown.

Shrimp in sweet chili sauce wrap
239 calories per serving

Very simple to make, the sweet chili sauce really adds a punch to this quick wrap.

Serves 1 Prep time: 2m

1 low-calorie tortilla
¼ cup shredded iceberg lettuce
3oz shrimp, cooked
1 tbsp sweet chili dipping sauce

Put the shrimp in a bowl with the chili sauce and mix thoroughly. Spread your lettuce over the wrap, leaving 1 inch at the bottom free. Place your prawn mixture over the lettuce, making sure the shrimp are near the middle but the sauce goes all over. Fold up the bottom inch and then roll carefully.

Roast chicken and pesto open flatbread
241 calories per serving

Serves 1 Prep time: 5m

1½oz ready-to-eat cooked roasted chicken (about ½ chicken breast)
2 tsp pesto
⅓ cup arugula or baby spinach
1 low calorie flatbread, such as Pepperidge Farm Deli Flats

Spread 1 teaspoon of pesto thinly over both halves of the flatbread. Spread the rocket leaves evenly over that. Cut the chicken into bite size pieces and mix the remaining pesto into the chicken. Spread the pesto chicken over the flatbread and grind some black pepper over the top.

Feta salad on toasted flatbread
260 calories per serving

Serves 1 Prep time: 5m Cook time: 5m

1oz reduced fat feta or Greek style cheese
1 tomato, diced
2 inches cucumber, diced
6 black olives pitted
2 basil leaves, torn
1 tsp extra virgin olive oil
1 tsp balsamic vinegar
freshly ground pepper
1 low calorie flatbread, such as Pepperidge Farm Deli Flats

Cut your feta into very small chunks and place in a bowl. Add in the tomato, cucumber and olives and mix. Toast your flatbread. Spread your salad equally over both slices of flatbread and drizzle over the olive oil and balsamic. Top with freshly ground pepper.

Chili chicken pita
273 calories per serving

Serves 1 Prep time: 5m Marinate time: 30m Cook time: 10m

2 spring onions, chopped finely
2 garlic cloves, chopped finely
juice ½ lemon
1 tsp honey
½ tsp paprika
¼ tsp mild chili powder
½ chicken breast fillet
1 pita bread
some iceberg lettuce

Mix together the spring onion, garlic, lemon juice, honey, paprika and chili powder. Cut the chicken into small lumps, no bigger than 1 inch square. Stir the chicken into the lemony marinade. Leave for at least half an hour.

Turn up your grill to the highest setting and when hot put your chicken on your grill pan and cook for about 4 minutes each side. They should be brown and crispy all over.

Toast your pitta. Cut in half and stuff with the chicken and shredded lettuce.

Mexican five bean wrap
294 calories per serving

This is the most filling lunch you can imagine; you won't need to eat for the rest of the day after this.

Serves 1 Prep time: 5m

1 reduced calorie tortilla
¼ 14oz canned mixed beans, drained
2 tablespoons grated light cheddar
1 tbsp salsa
shredded lettuce

Rinse and drain the beans. Spread the salsa evenly over the whole tortilla. Then add the beans, making sure you leave at least an inch free at the bottom of the wrap to fold over. Arrange your shredded lettuce over the beans and then sprinkle over the cheese as evenly as possible. Fold over the bottom inch of the wrap. Then gently but firmly roll up the wrap.

Soups

All the soups listed here (with the exception of the Ramen soup) make four to eight servings and can be frozen in individual portions.

Under 100 calories

Mushroom broth
44 calories per serving

Serves 4 Prep time: 5m Soak time: 10m Cook time: 30m

4 dried porcini mushrooms
1 cup brown mushrooms
4 cups vegetable or chicken stock
1 bay leaf
sprig fresh thyme
sprig fresh rosemary
3 leaves fresh parsley, chopped
3 tbsp sherry or Madeira (not cooking sherry!)

Firstly, place the porcini mushrooms in a cup and cover with boiling water. Leave to reconstitute for 10 minutes. Prepare the chestnut mushrooms by washing and then slicing. Put the chestnut mushrooms and stock in a large saucepan and bring to simmering point. Remove the porcini mushrooms from their soaking liquid and chop finely. Add to the pan, together with the soaking liquid, discarding the gritty dregs. Add the fresh herbs and simmer gently for ½ hour. Add the sherry or Madeira just before serving. Don't use cooking sherry – if you don't want to buy Sherry just for this recipe, a good substitute is a tablespoon of red wine vinegar mixed with a teaspoon of sugar.

Thai spinach soup
96 calories per serving

Serves 4 Prep time: 5m Cook time: 20m

1 tsp olive oil
1 medium onion, chopped
1 garlic clove, chopped
1 tsp ground cumin
4 cups of vegetable stock
1 tsp corn starch
⅓ cup reduced fat coconut milk
2 cups fresh spinach
1 tbsp green Thai curry paste
juice 1 lime

Heat the oil gently in a large saucepan and sauté the onions and garlic for 5 minutes. Stir in the cumin and add the stock. Now cover, bring to the boil and simmer for 15 minutes.

Mix the corn starch with a little water and add to the simmering stock, stirring well. Stir in the coconut milk, lime juice and Thai curry paste until dissolved. Add in the spinach and cook for one minute. Transfer to a blender and blend until smooth. Reheat gently in the pan.

Under 150 calories

Carrot and cilantro soup
111 calories per serving

I think this is my favorite warming winter soup. I just wish I could get my children to like it!

Serves 4 Prep time: 10m Cook time: 45m

1 tbsp vegetable oil
1 large onion, sliced
1lb carrots, peeled and sliced
1 tsp ground coriander
5 cups or 2 pints vegetable stock,
large bunch of fresh cilantro, roughly chopped

Heat the oil gently in a large pan and add the onions and carrots. Cook for 5 minutes until starting to soften. Stir in the ground coriander and season with salt and pepper. Cook for a further minute. Add the vegetable stock and bring to the boil. Simmer for 40 minutes. Use a blender to blend the soup until smooth. Reheat gently and stir in the fresh cilantro just before serving.

Garlic soup
121 calories per serving

Garlic soup is very warming and hearty. It is also exceptionally good for you.

Serves 6 Prep time: 10m Cook time: 1h

2 large heads of garlic
2 onions
1 tbsp olive oil
1 tbsp corn starch
6 cups of chicken/vegetable stock
1 tsp dried thyme
1 14oz can of cannellini beans, rinsed and drained
1 tbsp red wine vinegar

Separate the cloves of garlic, peel and slice. Chop the onion. In a large heavy saucepan, cook the garlic and onions in the oil on a very gentle heat. Stir often and cook for about 10 minutes until the onions are translucent. Stir in the corn starch and thyme and then immediately start adding the stock. Add the stock gradually to avoid lumps. Bring to the boil and simmer for 45 minutes.

Transfer the soup to a liquidiser (in small batches) and blend until smooth. Return to the heat and add the beans and red wine vinegar. Warm through and serve with black pepper.

Lentil, lemon and thyme soup
121 calories per serving

An easy soup from the pantry

Makes 4 generous servings Prep time: 5m Cook time: 45m

1 tbsp olive oil
1 large onion, finely diced
1 garlic clove, finely chopped
¾ cup red lentils, rinsed in a colander
2½ cups vegetable stock
1 14oz can of diced tomatoes
2 tsp tomato paste
2 tsp dried thyme, or 2 fresh sprigs
juice of ½ lemon

Heat the oil in a large saucepan and gently sauté the onions and garlic for 5 minutes until soft. Add the lentils and stir into the onions. Pour in the stock, then bring to the boil. Simmer vigorously for 10 minutes. Reduce the heat and add the thyme, diced tomatoes and tomato paste. Bring back to a quiet simmer and simmer gently for 30 minutes. Add the lemon juice and season to taste.

White Chicken Chili
128 calories per serving

A great alternative to the traditional bowl of red, with just the right level of spice and plenty of protein and complex carbs to keep you going. Leave out the jalapeno if you can't handle things too spicy – the canned green chiles are all flavor but no heat.

Makes 6 servings, can be frozen. Prep time: 15m Cook time: 20m

2 chicken breasts – about 4oz each
Small yellow onion, diced
2 cloves of garlic, chopped
1 fresh jalapeno, seeds and white membrane removed
4 sprays of olive oil cooking spray
14oz can of great Northern or cannellini beans
4 cups reduced-sodium chicken broth
2 4½oz cans of chopped green chiles
1 tsp ground cumin
1 tsp dried oregano
Salt and pepper
Fresh lime wedges and plain, fat-free yogurt to serve

Finely dice the onion, garlic, and jalapeno, and chop the chicken breast in to half-inch cubes. Spray a large, heavy-bottomed pot with the olive oils spray and sauté the chicken and diced ingredients over medium heat until the chicken is just cooked through. Add the beans along with their liquid, the chicken broth, the green chiles, the cumin, the oregano, and some black pepper. Bring to the simmer and taste for seasoning – there may be enough salt from the beans and chicken broth, but you can add a bit more if it's needed. Serve with a wedge of fresh lime and a tablespoon of plain, fat-free yogurt on top.

Under 200 calories

Savoy cabbage and bacon soup
156 calories per serving

Serves 4 Prep time: 10m Cook time: 25m

1 tbsp olive oil
1 onion, roughly chopped
1 garlic clove, roughly chopped
1 medium potato, peeled and roughly chopped
2½ cups chicken stock
½ savoy cabbage, shredded
4 pieces of turkey bacon
⅓ cup low-fat crème fraiche (or ⅓ cup low-fat plain yogurt)

Heat the oil in a large saucepan and gently sauté the onions and garlic for 5 minutes. Add the potato and stock, bring to the boil and simmer for 10 minutes. Add the cabbage and cook for a further 5 minutes.

Transfer to a blender (possibly in two batches) and blend until smooth. Re-heat the soup gently in the pan. In a separate frying pan, cook the bacon until crispy (4-5 minutes). Stir the crumbled bacon and crème fraiche or yogurt into the soup.

Pea and pesto soup
161 calories per serving

Serves 4 Prep time: 5m Cook time: 35m

1 tbsp olive oil
2 leeks, sliced
1 garlic clove, finely sliced
1 medium potato, peeled and diced
1 cup green peas, fresh or frozen
2 cups vegetable stock
¼ cup fava beans, fresh or frozen
1 cup baby spinach leaves
1 tbsp pesto

Heat the oil in a large saucepan and gently fry the leeks and garlic for 10 minutes. Add the potato, ¾ cup of the peas and the stock. Cover and simmer gently for 20 minutes.

Transfer the soup to a blender (possibly in two batches) and blend until smooth. Put the soup back in the pan and bring back to temperature. Stir in the rest of the peas, broad beans, spinach and pesto and season to taste. Bring to a gentle simmer and heat for a further 5 minutes.

Black-eyed pea and bacon soup
182 calories per serving

Serves 4 Prep time: 5m Cook time: 50m

4 pieces of turkey bacon, diced
1 14oz can black-eyed peas. rinsed and drained
1 medium onion, finely chopped
1 medium carrot, finely chopped
1 stick celery, finely chopped
4 cups chicken stock
2 cloves garlic, finely chopped
3 tbsp tomato paste
3 tsp hot sauce, or to taste
1 tsp dried oregano

In a large saucepan, cook the diced bacon and onion for about 4 minutes until the onion is translucent and the bacon is a little bit crispy. Then add the carrot, celery, garlic and chicken stock, stir and bring to the boil. Add the rest of your ingredients: black-eyed beans, tomato paste, hot sauce and oregano – and stir. Simmer gently for 45 minutes.

Spicy butternut squash soup
169 calories per serving

Serves 4 Prep time: 10m Cook time: 35m

1 tbsp olive oil
1 garlic clove, finely chopped
1 large or 2 small sweet potatoes (less than ½ pound total), peeled and diced
1 small butternut squash, peeled and diced
½ tsp smoked paprika
½ red chili, de-seeded and chopped
3½ cups vegetable stock
1 tbsp wholegrain mustard
1 tbsp parmesan cheese, finely grated
⅓ cup low-fat crème fraiche (or low-fat plain yogurt)

Heat the oil in a large saucepan or Dutch oven on the stovetop over low heat. Toss in the garlic, sweet potato and butternut squash. Stir, cover and cook gently for 10 minutes. Stir in the smoked paprika and red chili. Add the stock and bring to the boil. Cover and simmer for 20 minutes.

Remove from the heat and stir in the mustard and parmesan.

Transfer to a blender in two batches and blend until smooth. Return the soup to the pan and add the crème fraiche or yogurt. Reheat gently for 2 minutes and serve.

Chorizo and tomato soup
177 calories per serving

Makes 6 servings Prep time: 5m Cook time: 40m

1 tsp olive oil
1 onion, diced
1 garlic clove, finely sliced
1 green pepper, diced
3½oz of Spanish chorizo, diced (you can use Mexican chorizo, but as the Mexican version is a fresh sausage as opposed to a cured sausage, you'll want to add it in with the onion at the start of the recipe and cook until browned)
2 cups vegetable stock
1 14oz can diced tomatoes
1 14oz can tomato sauce
1 14oz can chick peas, rinsed and drained

Heat the oil in a saucepan, add the onion and sauté for 5 minutes. Add the garlic, green pepper and chorizo, then cook for a further 5 minutes. Add the stock, diced tomatoes, tomato sauce, and chick peas, then simmer for 30 minutes.

Red pepper soup with goat's cheese
192 calories per serving

Serves 6 Prep time: 10m Cook time: 35m

1 tbsp olive oil
1 large onion, roughly chopped
¾ cup red lentils, rinsed in a colander
8 cups vegetable stock
⅓ cup white wine
8 red peppers, de-seeded and roughly chopped
1 large cooking apple, peeled, cored and chopped
2 tsp dried basil
5oz rindless goat's cheese, roughly cut or broken up

Heat the olive oil gently in a large saucepan and sauté the onions for 5 minutes. Add the lentils, stir and pour in half the stock. Bring to the boil and simmer vigorously for 10 minutes. Then add the red peppers, apple, basil, white wine and the rest of the stock. Bring back to a gentle simmer and cook for a further 30 minutes.

Transfer to a blender – you'll need to do this in two or more batches – and blend until smooth. Return the soup to the pan and reheat gently. Stir in the goat's cheese until melted, then serve.

Under 300 calories

Ramen soup with udon noodles
215 calories per serving

This soup is incredibly satisfying and warming and can be made in under 10 minutes – and you can find the ingredients at most international or Asian groceries.

Serves 1 Prep time: 5m Cook time: 5m

2½oz frozen udon noodles or equivalent dry noodles cooked according to packet instructions
1 heaped tablespoon Miso soup paste
1 tsp mirin
1 tbsp dark soy sauce
½ inch fresh ginger, peeled and grated
1 cup spring greens or savoy cabbage, thinly sliced
½ carrot, cut into very fine batons
¼ cup beansprouts
½ cup Shiitake mushrooms, washed and sliced

Bring 2 cups water to boiling point in a saucepan. Stir in the miso paste, mirin, soy and ginger. Stir until the miso is dissolved. Add in the greens, carrot and mushrooms. Put the lid on the pan and simmer gently for 5 minutes.

In a separate pan pour boiling water over the noodles and simmer for 2 minutes. When they are warmed through drain and put them in a large soup bowl. Add the beansprouts to the ramen, stir and pour over the noodles. Drizzle a little good quality soy sauce over the top and serve.

Hearty ham soup
224 calories per serving

Two types of lentils plus the pearl barley make this a great recipe for a healthy heart.

Makes 4 servings Prep time: 10m Cook time: 1h 30m

1 tbsp olive oil
1 onion, finely diced
2 carrots, diced
¼ cup red lentils
¼ cup green puy lentils
¼ cup pearl barley
3 cups chicken stock
6oz cooked ham, cut into bite sized pieces
1 medium potato, peeled and diced

Heat the oil in a large saucepan and fry the onions and carrots very gently for 10 minutes until the onions are transparent.

Rinse the lentils and pearl barley, stir into the pan and then add the stock. Bring to the boil, cover and simmer for 45 minutes. Add the ham and potato and simmer for a further 30 minutes.

Vegetables

Under 100 calories

Roasted Broccoli
50 calories per serving

You will be amazed at how good this is – it has the power to convert vegetable-haters! Make a meal out of two servings with a poached egg on top for a very filling 170 calories.

Serves 4 very generously Prep time: 5m Cook time: 20m

1 pound fresh broccoli cut in to medium-sized florets
4 sprays of olive oil cooking spray
2 tsp freshly grated parmesan cheese
zest of one lemon (wash lemon in hot water and soap to remove wax)
plenty of salt and freshly ground black pepper

Preheat the oven to 450F. Steam broccoli using a stovetop or electric steamer, or in the microwave in a covered dish with a tablespoon of water, until just barely tender. You can boil it if you insist, but steaming – even in the microwave – is the best way to retain all the healthy vitamins.

Drain any liquid and let the broccoli sit uncovered for a couple of minutes to dry off a bit, and then toss with salt, pepper, parmesan, lemon zest, and two sprays of oil. Spray a baking sheet with the other two sprays of oil and spread the broccoli out in a single layer. Cook in the 450F oven for 15-20 minutes until the broccoli is blistered in places, with plenty of brown, crispy, roasty edges.

Under 200 calories

Garlic mushrooms
107 calories per serving

Serves 1 Prep time: 5m Cook time: 10m

2 large Portobello mushrooms
2 tsp extra virgin olive oil
1 garlic clove, finely chopped
1 tsp fresh parsley, finely chopped

Prepare the mushrooms by cleaning off any soil and cutting out the stalks. Cut the stalks up very small and mix in a small bowl with the oil, garlic and parsley. Place the mushrooms top side up on a baking sheet under a preheated broiler. Broil for 4 minutes. Take out the baking tray and turn the mushrooms over. Distribute the garlic and oil mixture evenly over the mushrooms. Sprinkle with salt and pepper. Place back under the broiler for a further 6 minutes. Serve immediately.

Ratatouille
155 calories per serving

Serves 1 Prep time: 10m Salting time: 1h Cook time: 35m

1 small eggplant
1 zucchini
1 tbsp salt
1 tsp olive oil
½ onion chopped
1 clove garlic chopped
½ red pepper, chopped
½ 14oz can diced tomatoes
Some chopped fresh basil if you have it

Wash and slice the eggplant and zucchini into ¼ inch slices. Quarter the eggplant slices. Put the eggplant and zucchini into a colander over a bowl. Add the salt and place a plate on the top plus something to weigh it down. Leave for about an hour and you should get some brown bitter juice coming out of the bottom. Wash in cold water before cooking.

In a pan with a lid, heat the olive oil and gently sauté the onion and garlic for about 5 minutes. Add the chopped pepper and the eggplant and zucchini. Add basil if you have it and some salt and pepper. Put the lid on and turn the heat to low and cook for 20 minutes. Add the diced tomatoes and heat gently for 10-15 minutes. Tastes even better if left to cool and then reheated.

Spinach and pea dahl
159 calories per serving

This is so tasty and filling that you really will forget you're on a diet.

Serves 4 Prep time: 10m Cook time: 50m

1 large onion
4 cloves garlic
1 inch thumb ginger
1 large red chili
1 tbsp sunflower oil
1¼ pint red lentils
¼ tsp turmeric powder
¼ tsp cayenne pepper
1 tsp paprika
½ tsp ground cumin
1 tsp salt
5 cups water
1 tomato
juice of 1 lime
2 tbsp frozen peas
½ cup frozen spinach, or 3 cups washed, drained, and chopped fresh spinach

Put the oil in a heavy bottomed pan over a low to medium heat.

Peel and roughly chop (or pulse in a food processor) the onion, garlic and ginger. Then coarsely chop the chili (removing the seeds and membrane if you don't want too much heat). Put all chopped ingredients into the pan and lightly sauté until the onion starts to turn translucent (about 5 minutes).

Once the onion has softened add all the ground spices, stir well and sauté for another minute or two.

Place the lentils in a fine colander and rinse under the cold tap for a minute. Next add the lentils to the pan and give the mixture a really good stir before adding all the water and turning the heat to high. Get the water at a fierce boil for ten minutes before turning it back down to low.

Now leave it on the lowest heat you can, stirring occasionally and watching that the dahl is not sticking on the bottom of the pan. Over the next 30 to 45 minutes it will thicken up considerably. Keep stirring occasionally until you have the consistency of thick oatmeal. Then add spinach, peas, lime juice and roughly chopped tomato and cook for a further five minutes (or another 10 minutes, if using fresh spinach) before serving.

Cauliflower curry
166 calories per serving

This curry is spicy but not hot.

Serves 2 Prep time: 10m Cook time: 25m

½ tsp ground cumin
½ tsp ground coriander
¼ tsp turmeric
1 tsp salt
juice ½ lemon
2 inch piece of fresh ginger, peeled and cut into matchsticks
1 tsp cumin seeds
½ tsp mustard seeds
1 tbsp peanut oil
2 tomatoes, diced
1 medium sized cauliflower, cut into small florets

First, mix all the ground spices and salt together in a small bowl. Add the lemon juice and 2 tbsp water.

In a large lidded frying pan heat the oil over medium heat. Quickly stir in the ginger and sauté for a minute before throwing in the cumin and mustard seeds. Cook for a minute and just as they start to sizzle and pop add in the cauliflower florets. Sauté for about 3-4 more minutes; you want to get brown spots appearing on the cauliflower.

Pour the spice and lemon juice mixture over the cauliflower, stir well, then turn the heat to low and put on the lid. Leave to steam for 8 minutes. Add the diced tomatoes, stir and cook for another 10-15 minutes until the cauliflower is tender.

Lemony leeks and mushrooms
179 calories per serving

One of my favorite suppers. Tasty, filling and easy.

Serves 1 Prep time: 5m Cook time: 12m

1 tbsp olive oil
3 medium leeks, cut into half-inch rings
2 cups chestnut mushrooms, washed and sliced
juice ½ lemon
freshly ground salt and pepper
sprinkling (teaspoon) of fresh-grated parmesan cheese

Heat the oil in a wide lidded frying pan or non-stick saucepan. Add in the leeks and fry on a medium heat for 5 minutes, stirring occasionally until the leeks have some brown bits. Add the mushrooms and continue to fry for a further 2 minutes.

Then add 2 tablespoons water, turn up the heat and put the lid on the pan. Cook for 5 minutes, then remove the lid. If there is any liquid remaining cook with the lid off until the water has boiled off. Remove from the heat and stir in the lemon juice. Serve in a wide bowl topped with salt, pepper and parmesan cheese.

Vegetable curry

181 calories per serving

You could use a pre-mixed madras curry powder instead of the spices. This could also be made in bigger portions and frozen.

Serves 1 Prep time: 5m Cook time: 40m

1 tsp sunflower oil
½ tsp cumin seeds
½ tsp mustard seeds
½ onion
1 clove garlic
¼ tsp ground coriander
¼ tsp ground cumin
¼ tsp turmeric
½ tsp mild chili powder
½ tsp salt
½ 14oz can of diced tomatoes
2 handfuls of pre-chopped frozen vegetables (California mix is good, but choose whatever you like!)

Finely chop the onion and garlic. In a deep wide frying pan heat the oil and whole spices (cumin and mustard seeds) together until the spices are just starting to pop. Add the chopped onion and garlic, stir and reduce the heat. Sweat the onions in the pan for up to 10 minutes until they are translucent. Add the ground spices and salt, then stir in thoroughly before adding the diced tomatoes. Add your choice of veggies and then simmer gently for ½ an hour.

Portobello mushrooms with spinach and tomato
195 calories per serving

The quinoa in this recipe adds good quality and filling protein. Who would believe this only has 195 calories?

Serves 1 Prep time: 5m Cook time: 15m

2 Portobello mushrooms
1½ cups washed, fresh (or ½ cup frozen) spinach
¾ cup pre-cooked quinoa or ⅛ cup dried quinoa cooked according to package
2 tsp light crème fraiche or low-fat plain yogurt
black pepper
1 tomato
½ clove garlic
1 tsp olive oil
1 tsp fresh grated parmesan

Remove the stalks from the mushrooms and set aside. Place the mushrooms on a baking sheet and bake for 8 minutes in a pre-heated oven at 400F.

Finely chop the mushroom stalks and dice the tomato. In a frying pan, gently heat the oil and sauté the mushroom stalks, garlic and tomato for 3-5 minutes. Then add the spinach, stir and warm through for 2 minutes. Remove from the heat. Stir in the quinoa and crème fraiche or yogurt. Pile the mixture onto the mushrooms and sprinkle with a little parmesan.

Place the mushrooms back in the oven and cook for a further 6-7 minutes, until the top is golden brown.

Under 300 calories

Sweet potato chili
212 calories per serving

Serves 4 Prep time: 5m Cook time: 1h 10m

1 tbsp vegetable oil
1 large onion, chopped
3 cloves garlic
2 fresh red or green chilis
2 large or 3 small sweet potatoes (about a pound in total), peeled and cut into big cubes
1 tsp mild chili powder
1 tsp ground cumin
2 tsp paprika
1 tsp cocoa powder
1 tsp salt
juice of 1 lime
1 14oz can diced tomatoes
1 14oz can red kidney beans

In a large Dutch oven or saucepan with a lid, gently sauté the onions for about 5 minutes. Chop and de-seed the chilis (to cut it into rounds: cut the top off, hollow out the seeds with an apple corer or the top of a potato peeler, then cut into circles.) Add the chilis and roughly chopped garlic to the onions and sauté for a further couple of minutes.

Add the sweet potato, stir in. Then add the chili powder, cumin, paprika, salt and cocoa and stir in. Finally add the canned tomatoes, kidney beans (including the water from the can) and lime juice. Stir well. Cook on the lowest heat for about an hour, lid on.

If you can, leave to cool completely before re-heating to serve – this really enriches the flavor.

Stuffed butternut squash
237 calories per serving

A tasty and filling low-calorie supper. Good for cold Autumn nights.

Serves 2 Prep time: 5m Cook time: 1 hour

3 tsp olive oil
1 butternut squash
1 white onion, chopped into fine half rings
½ red onion, chopped into fine half rings
1 inch thumb ginger
½ tsp cinnamon
½ tsp cumin seeds, crushed in a pestle and mortar
½ tsp paprika
1 tsp salt
2 tbsp golden raisins

Halve and de-seed the squash. Cut through the squash flesh almost to, but not through, the skin in two directions, about ½ inch apart, making squares or diamonds. Add 1 teaspoon of olive oil to each half and roast in the oven at 375F for 45 minutes.

Gently sauté both the red and white onion in the third teaspoon of oil for about 10 minutes. Remove from the heat. Chop the ginger into fine matchsticks and add to the onions. Add spices, salt and golden raisins to the onion mixture. Stuff the onions into the roasted squash halves and cook for a further 15 minutes.

One pot Thai curry
242 calories per serving

This is called a one pot curry because the rice is cooked within the recipe. I love to make this for dinner or lunch as it is so flavorsome and satisfying. As this makes six portions, there's plenty of opportunity to make a big pan and keep some (it freezes well) for another day.

Serves 6 Prep time: 10m Cook time: 40m

2 chilis, de-seeded and cut into fine rings
6 spring onions, chopped fine
1 inch thumb ginger, peeled and cut into matchsticks
pinch of mace
1 tsp salt
½ cup puy lentils
¾ cup brown rice
6½ cups chicken or vegetable stock
2 tbsp Thai green curry paste
1 small can water chestnuts drained and sliced
1 14oz can low-fat coconut milk
juice of 2 limes
2 cups beansprouts
4 cups fresh baby spinach

In a large saucepan place your chilis, spring onions, ginger, mace, salt, puy lentils and rice. Pour in your stock and bring to the boil. Stir in the green curry paste. Cook at a low simmer for 30 minutes, or until the lentils and rice is cooked through.

Now stir in the coconut milk and water chestnuts and simmer for another 5 minutes. Finally add in the beansprouts and spinach and add the juice of the limes, cook for 1-2 minutes, allowing the spinach to wilt and then serve.

One pot vegetable tagine
247 calories per serving

Like the Thai curry this is an all in one dish that really packs a punch.

Serves 6 Prep time: 10m Cook time: 30m

1 onion, sliced
1 carrot, chopped
4 cups chicken or vegetable stock
1 14oz can diced tomatoes
2 tsp mild chili powder
½ tsp cumin
1 tsp salt
¾ cup wild or red rice
8 dried apricots, chopped
½ cauliflower, chopped into small florets
1 14oz can chickpeas, drained
4 cups fresh, washed spinach

In a large Dutch oven or saucepan with a lid place your onions and carrots. Pour over your stock and bring to the boil. Pour in the rice and simmer vigorously for 10 minutes.

Next add the diced tomatoes, spices and salt and stir. Then add dried apricots, cauliflower and chickpeas. Bring back to a simmer and cook for a further 20 minutes. Check that your rice and cauliflower are both cooked through.

Add in the spinach and cook for 1 minute before serving.

Quinoa with red peppers
250 calories per serving

Serves 1 Prep time: 2m Cook time: 20m

1 red pepper, de-seeded and cut into long strips
¼ cup dried quinoa
1 tsp olive oil
½ onion, finely diced
1 garlic clove, finely sliced
1 bay leaf
½ tsp dried oregano
a little chopped fresh parsley if you have it

Put the pepper strips on a baking sheet and place under a pre-heated broiler for 5 minutes each side until tender and black at the edges. In a shallow pan heat the oil gently and sauté the onions and garlic for 10 minutes. Rinse the quinoa before stirring into the pan. Add the bay leaf and oregano. Add ½ cup water and simmer gently until the water is absorbed – about 8 minutes. Stir the peppers and parsley into the quinoa. Season with salt and pepper.

Broccoli with anchovy dip
251 calories per serving

Works with all kinds of broccoli, including the purple sprouting variety.

Serves 1 Prep time: 2m Cook time: 10m

1 cup broccoli, cut into florets, or about 6oz if you're using the long, thin stalk variety
1 tbsp olive oil
2 cloves garlic, very finely chopped or crushed
3 anchovy fillets, rinsed and dried

In a small saucepan heat a tiny bit of oil and gently sauté the garlic for 2 minutes. Then add the anchovy fillets and mash them slightly with the wooden spoon. Pour in the rest of the oil and cook over the lowest possible heat for another 6 minutes – if the garlic starts to get more than the lightest brown, remove it from the heat and let it cool for a few moments before continuing.

Meanwhile steam the broccoli for 6 minutes. Serve the dip warm in a small bowl surrounded by the broccoli.

Chicken

Under 200 calories

Herby chicken
185 calories per serving

This makes an extremely tasty and fresh dish. You could substitute the fresh herbs for ½ tsp of mixed dry herbs. Serve with a green vegetable such as broccoli or spinach.

Serves 1 Prep time: 5m Marinate time: 1h Cook time: 25m

1 5oz chicken breast
½ lemon
½ clove garlic (crushed)
salt and pepper to taste
mixed fresh herbs e.g. Rosemary, parsley or sage

Use a small oven proof and non-metallic dish that can hold the chicken breast with a little bit of space around it but not much more. Into your dish zest the lemon (wash in hot water and hand soap first if it is waxed) and then add the juice of half the lemon. Add your garlic and salt and pepper and then some roughly chopped herbs.

Snip or score the top of your chicken breast before adding it to the dish. Toss the chicken in the juices and herbs making sure it is covered. Leave it top side up and rub the herbs into the cuts in the chicken as much as you can. Cover with foil and leave to marinate for about an hour (at least ½ hour, but no more than three).

Cook in a pre-heated oven for 20 minutes at 360F, covered, and then uncover and cook at 450F for another 5 minutes.

Sticky Thai chicken
205 calories per serving

Serves 1 Prep time: 5m Marinate time: 1h Cook time: 10m

1 5oz chicken breast skinned and chopped into big chunks
1 clove garlic
1 small thumb ginger
1 tbsp soy sauce
½ tsp honey

Prepare the marinade by grating the garlic and ginger on the fine side of the grater. Mix in the soy sauce and honey. Add the chicken to the marinade and leave for at least one hour. Remove the chicken from the marinade and cook under a preheated broiler for 5-6 minutes, turning once, until cooked through. You can also thread the chicken chunks on a skewer and cook on the grill, away from direct heat.

Under 300 calories

Creamy chicken curry
245 calories per serving

Packed with flavor, this recipe serves 4 but can be frozen in batches.

Serves 4 Prep time: 10m Cook time: 55m

1 tbsp vegetable oil
1 tsp cumin seeds
¼ tsp black mustard seeds (if available)
2 onions, finely sliced
3 chicken breasts, cut into chunks
2 tsp turmeric
¼ tsp ground cinnamon
½ tsp ground ginger
½ tsp mild chili powder
1 tsp salt
1 14oz can diced tomatoes
½ cup water
3 cups baby spinach
2 tbsp mango chutney
4 tbsp light crème fraiche or low-fat plain yogurt

Heat the oil over medium heat in a Dutch oven or a saucepan with a lid. Add the cumin and mustard seeds and sauté for 1 minute or until they start to pop. Turn the heat down and add the onion, sauté gently for 5 minutes. Add in the rest of the spices and the salt, stir thoroughly. Add in the chicken and cook just until no longer pink, then add the diced tomatoes and water. Bring to the boil and then turn the heat back to simmer for 40 minutes.

Stir the spinach into the curry and cook for 1-2 minutes, allowing it to wilt. Stir in the mango chutney and crème fraiche. Warm through.

Chicken in tomato sauce
255 calories per serving

The tomato sauce is very versatile and can also be used on pasta and pizza. This recipe serves four but if you make the sauce for four you can keep or freeze some and use ¼ of the sauce with one chicken breast.

Serves 4 Prep time: 5m Cook time: 1h 10m

2 cloves garlic, finely sliced
1 tsp olive oil
2 14oz can of whole plum or roma tomatoes (not diced, if possible)
2 red peppers, de-seeded and chopped
1 zucchini, skinned and chopped
4 chicken breasts, skinless

In a wide saucepan gently heat the oil and toss in the garlic. Lightly sauté for 2-3 minutes. As the garlic is just starting to turn brown, add the tomatoes, peppers and zucchini. Bring to a simmer and then turn heat down as far as you can while still maintaining the barest simmer. Simmer like this for ½ hour, stirring occasionally. Then break up the tomatoes with a wooden spoon and continue to cook for a further ¼ hour.

To make a smooth sauce transfer to a blender and whizz for approx 1 minute. (You can of course skip this step and choose a more textured sauce.) In the same saucepan (or a smaller pan if you are just cooking one piece) place the whole pieces of chicken flat on the bottom of the pan. Pour over the sauce so it covers the chicken generously. Bring the sauce up to a simmer and cook for 25 minutes on a gentle heat until the chicken is cooked. If the pan looks dry or the chicken becomes uncovered you should add a little water and stir in.

Chicken with brown mushrooms
284 calories per serving

A lovely autumnal and earthy dish. Ideal served with ¼ savoy cabbage (27 calories).

Serves 1 Prep time: 5m Soak time: 30m Cook time: 15m

1 tsp olive oil
½ leek, chopped into rings
1 chicken breast cut into about 6 pieces
½ clove garlic
About 6 brown mushrooms, sliced
2 dried porcini mushrooms
1 tbsp sherry (if you don't want to buy a bottle, you can replace with a tablespoon of red wine vinegar mixed with a pinch of sugar)
1 tbsp light crème fraiche or plain, low-fat yogurt

Put the porcini mushrooms in a mug with ⅓ cup boiling water. Leave to soak for ½ hour. In a large frying pan heat the oil and fry the leeks and chicken on a medium heat for 8 minutes. Stir a few times but not too often.

Turn to a low heat and add the crushed garlic and brown mushrooms. Fry for 4 minutes.

Turn to a medium heat. Add the cooking sherry (it should sizzle a bit). Add the porcini mushrooms and the liquid you soaked them in, discarding the grit at the bottom of the cup. Add salt and pepper to taste. Simmer gently for 2 minutes before finally adding the crème fraiche or yogurt and serving.

Chicken with orange and black olives
284 calories per serving

Delicious served with a serving of spinach (14 calories for a ½ cup steamed portion).

Serves 1 Prep time: 5m Cook time: 15m

1 skinless chicken breast
¼ cup chicken stock
½ small orange
6 pitted black olives
pinch of dried sage
1 tsp olive oil

In a frying pan with a lid, gently heat the olive oil for a few minutes before adding the chicken breast. Cook for 2 minutes on each side on a medium to high heat. Turn the heat down and add the stock, the orange (quarter it, cut out the pith, cut the flesh out of the skin and roughly slice), olives and sage.

Put the lid on and cook for 10 minutes. Remove the lid and raise the temperature for 2 minutes to reduce the sauce a little.

Hot chicken curry
288 calories per serving

Serves 1 Prep time: 10m Marinate time: 30m Cook time: 1h

½ onion
1 clove garlic
1 chili
1 thumb ginger
1 skinless chicken breast
1 tbsp low fat yogurt
¼ tsp ground cumin
¼ tsp ground coriander
¼ tsp turmeric
½ tsp salt
¼ tsp garam masala
½ 14oz can diced tomatoes
a few sprays of olive oil cooking spray

Peel the onion, garlic and ginger, and de-seed the chili. Put all of them into a food processor and whizz until finely chopped. Place half the onion mix in a bowl and mix in the yogurt. Cube the chicken and add to the yogurt mixture. Leave for ½ hour.

Meanwhile in a Dutch oven or other oven proof pan, heat 3 or 4 sprays of olive oil spray over medium heat and add the rest of the onion mixture. sauté gently for 3 minutes, stirring now and again. Add all the spices and salt. In the processor (no need to clean after onions) whizz the tomatoes. Add the tomatoes to the pan and cook on lowest heat uncovered for ½ hour.

Add the chicken and yogurt to the pan, stir, and cover. Cook in preheated oven at 375F for 30 minutes.

Moroccan chicken casserole
291 calories per serving

An unusual and interesting mix of flavors. Ideal served with spinach (14 calories for a ½ cup steamed serving).

Serves 1 Prep time: 10m Marinate time: 2h Cook time: 25m

1 clove garlic
pinch of rock salt
½ tsp paprika
¼ tsp turmeric
¼ tsp cumin seed
1 chicken breast
1 tsp olive oil
½ onion
½ lemon
pinch saffron (optional)
5 green pitted olives

First you need to make a rub for the chicken. In a pestle and mortar, mash up the garlic with a pinch of rock salt and the cumin seeds. Then add the paprika and turmeric.

Score the chicken by cutting about ¼ inch into the surface in two directions, and then rub the mix all over the chicken. Leave for a few hours. 2 hours minimum, 4 ideal or even all day.

In a smallish lidded frying pan or saucepan sauté the finely sliced onions slowly in the oil for about 5 minutes uncovered. Remove the wax from the lemon by washing in hot water with soap. Cut four very thin slices of lemon. Layer the lemon on top of the onion and put the chicken breasts on top of that. Add enough water to just cover the chicken and bring to boil. Reduce to a low simmer and cook for 15 minutes with the lid on the pan.

Remove the chicken to a plate and cover to keep warm. Then remove the lid from the pan and increase the heat to high. Boil the liquid vigorously until it has reduced by half. This will take approximately ten minutes. Add the saffron and olives to the liquid and continue to cook for a further two minutes. Then serve the sauce poured over the chicken.

Jerusalem artichokes, leeks and chicken
294 calories per serving

Jerusalem artichokes are incredibly tasty and good for you. If you can get hold of them (normally best in October and November) this is my favorite recipe for them. Note that as the artichokes are quite substantial, I have reduced the amount of chicken.

Serves 2 Prep time: 10m Cook time: 15m

1 tbsp olive oil
6-8 Jerusalem artichokes
1 chicken breast, cut into small strips
1 large or 2 small leeks, cut into small rings.
juice of 1 lemon

First prepare your artichokes by cutting off the knobbly bits and then peeling. Cut into fine slices (not more than 2mm thick – a mandoline slicer is helpful!). Heat the oil on a high heat in a large lidded frying pan. Toss in the artichokes and sauté for 2 minutes.

Next add the leeks, turn the heat down, add 4 tablespoons water and place the lid on the pan. Cook for 6 minutes.

After this remove the lid from the pan and stir.

Turn the heat back up to medium high and when hot add the chicken pieces. Cook for another 5-6 minutes, stirring occasionally, until the chicken is cooked and all ingredients are browning nicely. Remove from the heat and stir in the lemon juice.

Fish

Under 200 calories

Classic British shrimp cocktail
160 calories per serving

This isn't the American version you're used to, with shrimp hooked over the side of a martini class filled with a horseradish and tomato sauce – this is the British version, which they (well, I!) call prawn cocktail. It's served with a creamy, tangy dressing.

Serves 1 Prep time: 5m

15 large shrimp, cooked
1 cup romaine hearts
2 inches cucumber, cut into chunky sticks
4 tsp extra light mayonnaise
1 tsp reduced sugar and salt ketchup
dash of Worcestershire sauce
1 tsp lemon juice
a little paprika

Mix together the mayonnaise, ketchup, Worcestershire sauce and lemon juice. Arrange the shrimp on a plate with the gem lettuce and cucumber. Serve the cocktail sauce in a small dish to dip, sprinkled with a little paprika.

Tilapia with a herb crust
185 calories per serving

Serves 2 Prep time: 5m Cook time: 12m

2 Tilapia fillets (approximately 4½oz each)
1 thin slice / ½ thick slice whole grain bread, crusts removed
1 lemon
2 tsp fresh herbs, shredded (oregano, parsley, basil or a mixture of all three)

Make breadcrumbs from the bread. Either blend in a food processor or chop into very small chunks with a bread-knife. Remove the wax from the lemon by washing in warm soapy water and dry. Finely grate the zest of the lemon into the breadcrumbs. Add in the fresh herbs and a little freshly ground salt and pepper. Stir in the juice of ½ lemon.

Put the fish fillets on a baking tray and gently press the bread-crumb mixture over the top. Cook in a pre-heated oven at 450F for 9-11 minutes. Serve on a bed of salad with a lemon wedge on the side.

Fresh pesto cod
187 calories per serving

Serve with fresh spinach, lightly cooked and drizzled with lemon juice and black pepper.

Serves 1 Prep time: 10m Cook time: 15m

1 skinless cod fillet, or another chunky white fish like basa
¼ cup fresh basil leaves
pinch of sea salt
1 tsp pine nuts
5g parmesan

Roughly chop your fresh basil. Place in a pestle and mortar with the sea salt and grind until you have a mushy paste. Add the pine nuts and pound again. Add a little water (2 teaspoons) and pound/stir once more. Spread the paste over your fish and place in an oven-proof dish. Grate a little (5g) parmesan over the top. Cook in a pre-heated oven at 220C (200C fan, 430F) for 15 minutes.

Fish sticks and salad
195 calories per serving

I know, I know, this is NOT a recipe. But the kids and I eat this quite happily at least twice a month. They just add ketchup. If you haven't eaten fish sticks in a while... try them, it should take you right back to childhood!

2 fish sticks
Standard salad (see page 45) including dressing

Under 300 calories

Coconut and cumin shrimp
206 calories per serving

This dish is also excellent made with crayfish if you can get hold of any. Serve with a salad of tomato, red onion, cilantro and lemon juice.

Serves 2 Prep time: 5m Cook time: 15m

1 tsp sunflower oil
½ tsp cumin seeds
½ onion, finely diced
2 tomatoes, diced
½ tsp salt
1 green chili, de-seeded and sliced
¼ tsp ground turmeric
¼ tsp mild chili powder
¼ 14oz can of low-fat coconut milk
½ pound raw shrimp, shelled (defrosted if frozen)

Heat the oil on a medium heat in a wide, lidded frying pan. When it's hot toss in the cumin seeds and when they are sizzling add in the onion and stir. Sauté gently until golden – about 5 minutes.

Turn the heat to low. Add the tomatoes, salt, chili, ground turmeric and chili powder. Stir well. Gently cook for 5 minutes. Stir in the coconut milk, heat for another 3 minutes. Stir in the shrimp, and finally cook with the lid on for another 3 minutes.

Cajun salmon
213 calories per serving

A simple way to jazz up a piece of salmon. Serve with a salad.

Serves 1 Prep time: 1m Cook time: 15m

1 skinless salmon fillet
1 tsp Tony Chachere's Creole seasoning

Pre-heat oven to 450F. Place the salmon fillet on a baking sheet.
Rub a teaspoon of cajun spices over the fillet. Cook for 15
minutes.

Chunky cod with tomatoes and spinach
248 calories per serving

Serves 2 Prep time: 10m Cook time: 20m

2 cod fillets, skinless (about 4½ ounces each) or another white fish like basa or
orange roughy
sea salt crystals
2 tsp olive oil
2 tbsp capers
3 tomatoes, diced
½ onion
1 clove garlic, finely chopped
pinch chili flakes
2 cups baby spinach

Cut each piece of cod into 3 pieces. Rub a little of the sea salt
onto each of the cod chunks. Heat 1 tsp oil in a small frying pan
and add the capers. Fry for 4-5 minutes until they turn crispy but
not burnt. Heat the remaining teaspoon of oil in pan with a lid.
Add the onion and garlic and cook over a low heat for 10 minutes
until translucent.

Add the chili flakes and tomato, stir, and lay the cod pieces on top with a scattering of freshly ground pepper.

Place the lid on the pan and steam the fish for 10 minutes.

When the fish is cooked, remove it from the pan and set aside. Put the spinach into the pan, stir and put the lid on. Leave to wilt for 1-2 minutes. Then stir again, transfer to plates and put the cod on the top. Scatter over the crispy capers.

Salmon and cod fishcakes
256 calories per serving

Serves 4 Prep time: 10m Cook time: 40m

2 skinless salmon fillets
1 skinless cod fillet, or other chunky white fish like basa or orange roughy
1 bay leaf
a little dill
1 cup dry white wine
⅓ cup light mayonnaise
½ cup breadcrumbs

Place the fish in a baking dish with the bay leaf and dill. Pour over the white wine and cover with foil. Cook in a pre-heated oven at 375F for 22 minutes. Allow to cool and drain and dry on some kitchen paper.

Using a fork, break up the fish into smaller pieces. Then add in the breadcrumbs, mayonnaise and some salt and pepper. Combine thoroughly. Shape the fish mixture into balls, making 12-14 in total. Place the balls on a non-stick baking tray and flatten into cakes with the palm of your hand.

Cook in a pre-heated oven at 425F for 12-15 minutes until starting to brown.

Scallops with garlic tomatoes
258 calories per serving

Serves 1 Prep time: 5m Cook time: 10m

¾ cup fresh green beans
6 cherry tomatoes, halved
1 tsp olive oil
1 clove garlic, very finely sliced
3½oz scallops

Cook the green beans by boiling in water for 4 minutes. In a frying pan gently heat the oil. Toss in the garlic and after 1 minute add the cherry tomatoes. Sauté gently for 4 minutes. Remove tomato mixture from the pan and turn the heat up to medium high. Cook the scallops for 30 seconds to 1 minute each side until opaque and just cooked through.

Put the green beans on a warm plate and arrange the scallops over the top. Scatter with black pepper. Finally place the tomatoes and garlic on the top.

Oven baked tandoori salmon
281 calories per serving

Serve with broccoli or peas.

Serves 1 Prep time: 5m Marinate time: 1h Cook time: 15m

1 skinless salmon fillet
¼ cup low fat plain yogurt
juice of half lemon
1 small thumb ginger
1 clove garlic
½ tsp ground cumin
½ tsp chili powder
¼ tsp turmeric
¼ tsp garam masala
½ tsp salt

Grate the ginger and garlic on the fine side of the grater. Mix all the ingredients except the salmon together. Put the salmon in a plastic bag and mix in the yogurt paste. Marinate for an hour. Shake off the excess marinade and cook in a preheated oven at 425F for 15 minutes.

Spicy Indian shrimp and rice
290 calories per serving

Serves 2 Pre-time: 5m Cook time: 25m

⅓ cup basmati rice (dry measure)
2 tsp sunflower oil
¼ tsp cumin seeds
½ cinnamon stick
2 cloves
1 bay leaf
½ onion, finely chopped
1 birds eye chili, de-seeded and sliced
4 cloves garlic, finely chopped
½ tsp mild chili powder
1 tsp paprika
½ tsp salt
2 fresh tomatoes, diced
5oz cooked shrimp

Cook the rice by your preferred method and leave to cool.

Heat the oil in a wide frying pan on medium high heat. Add the cumin seeds, bay leaf, cinnamon and cloves. Sauté for 1 minute before adding the chopped onion, chili and garlic. Sauté gently for 5 minutes until the onions are starting to brown.

Add the tomatoes, chili powder, paprika and salt. Continue cooking on a low heat for a further 7 minutes. Add the shrimp and rice and cook gently for 5 more minutes until they are warmed through.

Catfish with olives and tomatoes
293 calories per serving

Serve with green beans or spinach.

Serves 1 Prep time: 2m Cook time: 12m

1 good-sized skinless, boneless catfish fillet
1 tbsp black olive paste or meze
1 tsp extra virgin olive oil
4 cherry tomatoes, quartered
2 basil leaves, shredded
juice of ½ lime

Spread the olive paste on both sides of the fish. Heat a non-stick frying pan on a medium high heat and place the fish in the pan. Cook for 7-10 minutes, turning once. The cooking time depends on the thickness of the fillet. Remove the fish to a warm plate. Add the tomatoes, olive oil, basil and lime juice to the pan. Heat for 2 minutes and serve poured over the fish.

Steamed salmon with Chinese vegetables
296 calories per serving

Serves 1 Prep time: 10m Cook time: 10m

¼ onion, thinly sliced
1 salmon fillet, skinless and boneless
¼ savoy cabbage, sliced
½ small carrot (cut into small strips)
½ fennel bulb (cut into small strips)
1 small thumb ginger, grated
1 tbsp Soy sauce
2 drops nam pla (Fish sauce)
2 drops Sesame oil

In a large frying with a lid add about ¼ inch depth of water and bring to a boil. Add the onion, carrot and fennel and put the lid on. Continue on full heat for 5 minutes. Check water level and add the cabbage. Put the lid back on and cook for a further 5 minutes over medium high.

Add the grated ginger, soy and fish sauce and stir in. If necessary add a little more water too. Cut the salmon into big chunks and place on top of the veg. Add the 2 drops of sesame oil. Put the lid back on and steam for 6 minutes. Serve carefully to stop the salmon breaking up.

Haddock with Sauce Vierge
300 calories per serving

Serves 2 Prep time: 15m Cook time: 20m

*2 haddock fillets, skinless and boneless, or another white fish like basa or orange
roughy – about 4½ ounces each*
2 tbsp extra virgin olive oil
½ tsp ground cumin
½ tsp ground coriander
3 sprigs saffron
1 red pepper, de-seeded and finely chopped
1 tomato, finely chopped
1 tsp fresh mint, finely shredded
1 tsp fresh coriander, finely shredded

Place the saffron in a small cup or bowl and pour over a small
amount of boiling water. Leave to steep for 10 minutes.

Heat a small frying pan to a medium high heat. Put the red
peppers in the frying pan with no oil. Chargrill the red peppers for
about 4 minutes each side. They should be tender and a little
black on the outside.

Put the haddock fillets on a baking tray and sprinkle with salt and
pepper. Bake in a pre-heated oven at 400F for 15-18 minutes
until cooked through.

In a small saucepan combine the olive oil, spices, saffron
(including the soaking liquid), cooked red pepper, tomato and
fresh herbs. Heat for two minutes very gently until the sauce is
warm but not too hot. Serve poured over the baked fish.

Teriyaki salmon
310 calories per serving

Flavorsome one-dish meal.

Serves 1 Prep time: 5m Marinate time: 2h Cook time: 15m

1 skinless salmon fillet
1 inch thumb ginger, grated
1 clove garlic, grated or crushed
1 tsp nam pla or fish sauce
1 tsp soy sauce
½ tsp sesame oil
1 tsp honey
½ cup water
1 head of bok choy, chopped
6 mushrooms, sliced
¼ savoy cabbage, finely sliced

First make your marinade by mixing together the ginger, garlic, nam pla, soy sauce, sesame oil, honey, and water. Put the marinade in a wide bowl. Put the salmon in the bowl and scoop up some of the marinade to cover all the salmon. Leave for about 2 hours.

Cook your salmon on a grill pan over medium high heat, or away from direct heat on an outdoor grill, for about 5 minutes on each side until golden brown and cooked through. Save the marinade for cooking the vegetables.

To prepare the bok choy, mushrooms and cabbage, pour the extra marinade into a wide saucepan with a lid. Heat the marinade on high with the lid on for several minutes until it reaches a hard boil. Add in your chopped vegetables and stir. Quickly replace the lid and steam over medium heat for 5 minutes.

Meat

Under 200 calories

Pork tenderloin with peaches and thyme
160 calories per serving

This is a great recipe to serve when you have unavoidable guests on a fast day. Serve with roasted broccoli (pg 80), along with some mashed potatoes for the non-dieters

Serves 4 Prep time: 5m Cook time: 25m

1 pound pork tenderloin, with as much visible fat removed as possible
1 no-added-sugar single-serving cup of diced peaches, such as Del Monte Fruit Naturals, or – if in season – two small peaches, peeled and diced, plus two tablespoons of water
1 teaspoon whole grain mustard
½ tablespoon fresh thyme leaves (no need to chop, just pull the leaves off of the woody stem and crush slightly with the flat side of a knife)
4 sprays of olive oil cooking spray
Salt and pepper

Preheat the oven to 400F. Season the pork with salt and pepper, spray an oven-safe skillet with the cooking spray, and brown the tenderloin on each side on the stovetop over medium-high heat. Once the tenderloin has a nice brown sear, put the skillet in the oven to finish cooking for 12 minutes, or until a meat thermometer in the thickest part of the tenderloin registers 140F. Remove the tenderloin to a plate to rest, covered loosely in foil, while you make the sauce.

Put the skillet back over medium heat on the stovetop. Add the peaches along with the juice (or water, if using fresh peaches) to the skillet, and stir vigorously with a heat-proof spatula to scrape up all the delicious brown bits in the pan. Add the thyme and mustard and season with salt and pepper to taste. If the sauce seems to thick or dry, just add a little water.

Slice the tenderloin into thin medallions, and serve with the sauce spooned over top.

Kale with bacon and tomato
197 calories per serving

Easy to rustle up, this is warming and filling.

Serves 1 Prep time: 5m Cook time: 20m

2 sprays of olive oil cooking spray
½ onion, diced
2 pieces of turkey bacon
¼ 11oz can haricot or navy beans
1 tomato, diced
4 packed cups (or as much as you can fit in the pan) of curly leaf kale

In a wide saucepan with a lid, sauté the onion slowly in the spray oil for 5 minutes. Then turn the heat up to medium and add the bacon. Cook for a further 5 minutes, turning now and again. Now add the beans, tomato and 3 tablespoons water. Stir and then add the kale on the top. Put the lid on the pan, turn the heat up high and cook for 6-8 minutes until the kale is cooked through and tender.

Autumn lamb stew
198 calories per serving

The following recipe serves eight people. It is therefore suitable for cooking in bulk and freezing in individual portions.

Serves 8 Prep time: 15m Cook time: 2h 30m

1 pound lean diced lamb
2 tbsp olive oil
1 onion
2 carrots
4 celery stalks
2 cloves garlic
1 cup red wine
1 small turnip
2 tbsp tomato paste
2 14oz cans diced tomatoes
2 bay leaves
2 cups vegetable or chicken stock

Heat the oil in a Dutch oven or a large, oven-safe saucepan with a lid (you can also transfer to a slow cooker). Add the lamb and roughly chopped onions. Cook for 5 minutes until the lamb starts to brown. Roughly chop all the other vegetables (this is a big chunky stew). Add the sliced garlic and chopped veggies. Stir and cook for another 5 minutes.

Add the rest of the ingredients and bring to the boil. Simmer gently for 30 minutes. Either transfer to a slow cooker for about 8 hours or cook with the lid on for about 4 hours at 140C (120C fan, 275F) or 2 hours at a very low simmer.

Kofta lamb meatballs
200 calories per serving

This would also be tasty with extra lean ground beef, but seek out the ground lamb for a really authentic Greek dish. If you have a local butcher that carries lamb, they will be able to grind a lean cut of lamb for you. Serve on a bed of crispy salad leaves with a wedge of lemon.

Serves 4 Prep time: 10m Cook time: 20m

¾ pound extra lean ground lamb
1 onion, peeled and chopped
2 tsp ground cumin
2 garlic cloves, peeled
pinch cayenne pepper
handful of fresh cilantro leaves
1 tsp baking powder
1 tsp salt
1 tbsp olive oil

Place all the ingredients except the olive oil in a food processor and blend. The mixture needs to be sticking together but not smooth.

Take a small handful of the mixture and make into a small oval ball (the kofta). The mixture should make about 16 koftas. Brush each kofta with a little olive oil and place on a non-stick baking tray. Pre-heat the oven to 375F and cook for 20 minutes until brown and crispy.

Under 300 calories

Honey mustard pork chop
228 calories per serving

Serve with a green vegetable such as broccoli, green beans or spinach.

Serves 1 Prep time: 2m Cook time: 15m

1 lean, trimmed boneless pork chop (about 4½ ounces)
salt and pepper
1 tsp honey
½ tsp English mustard powder
1½ tsp red wine vinegar
½ tsp ketchup
2 tbsp water

Season the pork with salt and pepper. Heat a frying pan to a medium heat and add the pork chop. You want it to be just sizzling the whole time. Cook for approximately 7 minutes each side.

Meanwhile make the sauce by simply mixing the rest of the ingredients together in a small bowl. Add a generous quantity of salt and pepper to the sauce as well.

When you are happy that the pork is well cooked (you can use a meat thermometer to check for a temperature of 140F, or cut into the center with a small, sharp knife to ensure it's just barely pink if you're not sure) turn the heat to low and pour in the sauce over the pork. It should sizzle frantically at first and then calm down to a gentle bubble. Cook for a further minute or two.

Fried pork tenderloin sandwich with sweet and sour coleslaw
230 calories per serving

A fried pork tenderloin sandwich with a side of coleslaw for under 250 calories? Believe it! Add some potato salad from the deli counter to make it a hearty meal for the non-dieters at your table.

Serves 4 Prep time: 15m Marinating time: 30 minutes Cook time: 15m

Make the slaw first:
½ medium white cabbage
1 carrot
½ cup apple cider vinegar
½ cup water
1 tsp mustard seeds
1 tbsp brown sugar
1 tsp salt

Using a grater or food processor, shred the cabbage and carrot together into a glass or stoneware bowl. Bring the rest of the ingredients to the boil on the stovetop and pour over the cabbage and carrot mixture. If it doesn't completely cover, boil some more water to top it up. Let it marinate while you prepare the sandwiches.

For the sandwiches:
½ pound pork tenderloin, cut in to eight medallions. Use a very sharp knife to get clean slices
2 tbsp plain flour
salt and pepper
8 sprays of ollive oil cooking spray – 4 sprays for each batch of four medallions
Pepperidge Farm Deli Flat rolls to serve

Place the medallions one at a time between two sheets of plastic wrap, and pound with a wooden rolling pin until they are 30-40% bigger than when you started. Mix the flour with some salt and pepper in a dish and dredge the pork medallions, shaking off any excess. Heat a large non-stick skillet over medium low heat with the cooking spray and fry the pork in two batches until browned and cooked through. The trick to frying in a tiny amount of oil is to keep the heat low and use a good-quality non-stick pan – but if you can't get them as brown as you'd like, a minute or two under the broiler will crisp them up nicely.

Serve two medallions on a roll for each person with a bit of mustard, and the slaw either on the sandwich or next to it.

Quick fried steak with Salsa Verde
224 calories per serving

Eye of round steak is much less expensive than fillet mignon, is easy to cook and has only 160 calories per serving. Try serving with green beans.

Serves 2 Prep time: 10m Infuse time: 15m+ Cook time: 5m

2 leaves flat leaf parsley
2 basil leaves
2 mint leaves
1 large/ 2 small sweet pickles
1 garlic clove, peeled
1 tsp capers
2 anchovy fillets
1 tsp red wine vinegar
juice of ½ lime
1 tsp Dijon mustard
1 tsp extra virgin olive oil
2-3 sprays of olive oil cooking spray
2 lean eye of round beef steaks (up to 4½ ounces each)

Coarsely chop the herbs, pickles, garlic and anchovy fillets. Place in a bowl with the capers. Add in the red wine vinegar, lime juice, mustard and olive oil. Add in a tablespoon of water and some ground black pepper. Stir and set aside (the flavors develop best if left for up to an hour).

Heat a heavy based frying pan (cast iron is best for steaks!) over medium high heat. Spray the pan with a little olive oil cooking spray, add in your steaks, seasoned with salt and pepper, and cook for 2-3 minutes each side, depending on how you like your steak.

Lamb tagine
227 calories per serving

This Moroccan-inspired tagine (stew) is a favorite in our house.

Serves 8 Prep time: 15m   Cook time: 2h 45m

2 tbsp oil
1¼ pound extra lean diced lamb – ask your butcher for a lean cut that's good for slow-cooking.
1 large / 2 small onions, sliced
2 garlic cloves, finely sliced
2 sticks celery, diced
1 carrot, diced
4 sun-dried tomatoes, re-hydrated in boiling water if dried
2 tsp mild chili powder
½ tsp cumin powder
2 tsp salt
1 14oz can diced tomatoes
1 14oz can chickpeas, drained
8 dried apricots chopped
12 black pitted olives
juice of 1 lime
juice of 1 lemon

Heat the oil in a large Dutch oven or a heavy, oven-safe pan with a lid and sear the lamb in 2 batches. Cook for 2 minutes each side until it starts to get brown and crispy. Remove the lamb to a plate and set aside.

Reduce the heat in the pan and add the onions and garlic. Cook slowly for 5 minutes. Add the carrot and celery and continue heating slowly for another 5 minutes. Stir in the spices and salt. Put the meat back in the pan. Then add the tomatoes, chickpeas, apricots and olives. Bring up to simmer and cook with the lid off for ½ hour.

Put the lid on and cook in the oven for 2 hours at 350F or for 8 hours in a slow cooker. At the end of the cooking time, stir in the lemon and lime juice.

Chili con carne
235 calories per serving

This chili tastes even better if chilled or frozen and re-heated.

Serves 8 Prep time: 10m Cook time: 2h 30 minimum

1 tsp sunflower oil
1 large onion (or 2 small) chopped
3 cloves garlic, roughly chopped
2 fresh green or red chilis
2 pounds extra lean ground beef
1 tsp mild chili powder
1 tsp ground cumin
2 tsp paprika
1 tsp cocoa powder
1 tsp salt
juice of 1 lime
1 14oz can diced tomatoes
1 14oz can red kidney beans

In a large Dutch oven or heavy-bottomed saucepan gently sauté the onions in the oil for about 5 minutes, until translucent. Chop and de-seed the chilis.

Add the chilis and garlic to the onions and fry for a further couple of minutes. Add the ground beef and continue frying until browned. Then add the chili powder, cumin, paprika, salt and cocoa. Finally add the lime juice, canned tomatoes and kidney beans. Stir well and simmer gently for 30 minutes.

Add a little water if it looks like it might dry out during cooking. Transfer to a slow cooker for about 8 hours, oven-cook for about 4 hours at 275F, or on the stovetop for 2 hours at a very low simmer. If cooking on the stovetop, check frequently to make sure it's not sticking and burning.

Texas chili beef stew
238 calories per serving

The following recipe serves eight people – great for cooking in bulk and freezing in individual portions.

Serves 8 Prep time: 10m Cook time: 2h 30 minimum

2 tbsp sunflower oil
2 pounds lean diced stewing beef
1 tsp red chili flakes
1 tsp ground cumin
2 tsp paprika
1 tsp salt
3 cloves garlic – finely chopped
1 14oz can diced tomatoes
1 butternut squash, peeled and diced
1 sweet potato, peeled and diced

Toss the chopped beef in the spices and seasoning until it is well covered. Heat the oil in a large oven-proof saucepan and wait until it is really hot. Add the beef to the saucepan and brown all over. You may have to do this in 2 batches. It is likely to stick to the bottom but don't worry!

Add the chopped garlic and fry for another minute. Add the tinned tomatoes and the veg and bring to simmering point. Simmer gently for 30 minutes. Add a little water if it looks like it might dry out during cooking.

Transfer to a slow cooker for about 8 hours, oven-cook for about 4 hours at 275F, or on the stovetop for 2 hours at a very low simmer.

Steak in mushrooms and wine
294 calories per serving

Serve with any green vegetable.

Serves 2 Prep time: 5m Cook time: 25m

4 dried porcini mushrooms
1 tsp vegetable oil
1 onion, finely diced
1 garlic clove, finely chopped
8 brown or white mushrooms, washed and sliced
1 cup red wine
1 tsp corn starch
2 lean eye of round beef steaks (up to 4½ ounces each)

Put the porcini mushrooms in ¼ cup of boiling water and leave to soak for at least 15 minutes. In a frying pan heat the oil over medium-low heat and add the onions. Cook gently for 10 minutes. Add the sliced mushrooms and garlic and cook gently for a further 5 minutes. Remove the mushroom mixture from the pan and set aside.

Turn up the heat to medium high and sear the beef for about 1 minute each side. Reduce the heat and reintroduce the mushroom mix. Stir in the red wine. Finely slice the porcini mushrooms and add them, together with their soaking liquid. Bring the mixture to a gentle simmer. Mix the corn starch with a little water and add to the pan. Stir well. Simmer for 5-10 minutes.

Paprika pork casserole
307 calories per serving

This recipe makes eight portions. It is suitable for freezing.

Serves 8 Prep time: 10m Cook time: 2h 30 minimum

2 tbsp oil
2 pounds diced lean pork shoulder
1 large onion
2 peppers (red, yellow or green)
2 cloves garlic, chopped
1 tsp hot paprika
1 tsp smoked paprika
2 14oz cans diced tomatoes
1 tsp salt
1 chicken stock cube
¾ cup light crème fraiche or low-fat plain yogurt

Toss the pork in some salt and pepper. In a Dutch oven or another oven-safe pan with a lid, fry off the pork in small batches in very hot oil and set aside when starting to turn brown.

Roughly chop the onion and sauté gently in the left over oil for about 5 minutes.

Then add the peppers, garlic and the meat. Stir in the 2 types of paprika and then add the tinned tomatoes, crumbled stock cube and a little salt. Simmer gently for 30 minutes. Add a little water if it looks like it might dry out during cooking.

Transfer to a slow cooker for about 8 hours or else cook in the oven with the lid on for about 4 hours at 275F or on the stove top for 2 hours at a very low simmer. Stir in the crème fraiche or plain yogurt before serving.

Sweet treats

Under 150 calories

Chocolate dipped strawberries
90 calories per serving

Makes 4 servings Prep time: 10m Chilling time: 30m

8oz strawberries
2oz dark 70% chocolate

First remove the stalks from the strawberries, halve any big ones, wash them and dry on some paper towels. Prepare a large plate or baking tray by covering it with wax paper.

Break the chocolate into chunks and put into a small heat proof bowl. Place the bowl over a saucepan of simmering water. Stir occasionally and when the chocolate has completely melted move the pan and bowl together to where you want to dip your strawberries.

You can also melt the chocolate in the microwave on high, 10 seconds at a time, until it looks glossy, and then 5 seconds at a time until it's about 80% melted. You can finish melting from this point by stirring with a small spoon.

Hold the fat end of a strawberry and dip the tip into the melted chocolate. You want the strawberry to be about one third covered. Then place the strawberry, tip up (if possible!) on the wax paper. Repeat with all the strawberries. Place the strawberries in the fridge to set.

Meringues with strawberry compote
100 calories per serving

Trader Joe's Vanilla Meringues are fat free and have only 25 calories each! If you're not near a Trader Joe's, have a look in the healthy treats section of your local grocery to find meringues with a similar amount of calories. The strawberry compote lasts for up to 3 days covered in the fridge.

Makes 4 servings of compote

8oz strawberries
2 tbsp granulated sugar
juice of 1 lemon

2 meringues per person

Hull and wash the strawberries. Cut into thin slices (2-4mm). Place the strawberries in a bowl and cover with sugar. Squeeze over the lemon juice and stir in well. Leave for at least ½ hour for the flavors to combine.

Serve chilled poured over the meringues.

Apricot cereal bars
139 calories per serving

Finding a snack to eat on the go can be a real challenge. These apricot cereal bars are nutritious and sustaining. They also keep for up to 2 weeks in an air-tight container. An individual slice can easily be wrapped in plastic wrap for eating wherever and whenever.

Makes 16 servings Prep time: 10m Cook time: 45m

1 can fat-free sweetened condensed milk
2½ cups rolled oats
1 cup dried apricots
2-3 sprays of oil spray

Line an 8" non-stick square cake pan with baking parchment and spray with olive oil cooking spray to prevent sticking. In a small pan, warm the condensed milk on a low heat for about 5 minutes. You want it to be warm but not boiling.

Meanwhile, chop the apricots into small pieces and mix into the oats in a large mixing bowl.

When the condensed milk has just started to steam, pour it in over the oats and apricots and mix thoroughly. Scoop this mixture into your cake tin and bake in a pre-heated oven at 325F for 45 minutes.

When you remove the tin from the oven, immediately transfer the cooked bars to a cutting board and cut into 16 squares with a very sharp knife. Then leave to cool completely on the cutting board before storing in an air-tight container.

Calorie counting reference

Although by no means extensive this covers a lot of the food that you are likely to eat on your diet days.

Lower calorie carbs

Couscous	¼ cup serving (dry weight)	160 calories
New potatoes	6 ounces – about 4 medium new potatoes	135 calories
Pita bread	½ pita	80-100 calories
Crispbread	2 pieces	60 calories
Quinoa	¼ cup serving (dry weight)	140 calories
Tortilla (low-calorie)	1 Tortilla	80 calories
White, jasmine, or Basmati rice	¼ cup serving (dry weight)	141 calories

Meat, fish and eggs

Egg	1 large egg	70 calories
Egg white	1 egg white	18 calories
Chicken	1 chicken breast, without skin (approximately 6oz)	175 calories
Salmon	1 avg salmon fillet, skin off (approximately 4oz)	200 calories
Tilapia or Basa filet	1 avg filet (approximately 4oz)	113 calories
Extra lean ground beef	½ cup – (approximately 4 ½oz)	190 calories
Lean, boneless pork loin chop	1 pork chop (approximately 4½oz)	276 calories

Calorie counting reference

Beef eye of round steak	1 steak (approximately 4oz)	170 calories
Cod	1 cod fillet (approximately 4½oz)	127 calories
Shrimp	1 portion (2½oz)	60 calories

Vegetables and salad

Lettuce	¼ iceberg lettuce	14 calories
Cucumber	3½oz (2 inches, 5cm)	10 calories
Tomato	2 medium tomatoes	44 calories
Broccoli	3½oz serving	33 calories
Savoy Cabbage	3½oz serving, ¼ cabbage	27 calories
Onion	1 med onion, 6½oz	55 calories
Red pepper	1 med pepper, 3½oz	32 calories
Green pepper	1 med pepper, 3½oz	15 calories
Mushrooms	1 serving, 3½oz	13 calories
Leeks	1 serving, 3½oz	23 calories
Bok Choy	1 serving, 3½oz	11 calories
Kale	1 serving, 2oz	16 calories
Spinach	1 serving, 2oz	14 calories
Peas	1 serving, 3oz	54 calories
Zucchini	1 med zucchini 5oz	33 calories
Green beans	1 serving, 3½oz	35 calories

Other

| Canned beans – kidney, white, or chickpeas | ¼ can (3½oz) | 80-100 calories |
| Canned tomatoes | ½ can (7oz) | 42 calories |

Sources & bibliography

Healthy fellow interview with Dr Krista Varady

http://www.healthyfellow.com/511/alternate-day-fasting-interview-part-1/

http://www.healthyfellow.com/517/dr-krista-varady-interview-part-2/

The American Journal of Clinical Nutrition "Alternate Day Fasting and Chronic Disease Prevention: A Review of Animal and Human Trials"

http://ajcn.nutrition.org/content/86/1/7.full

The power of intermittent fasting

http://www.bbc.co.uk/news/health-19112549

The American Journal of Clinical Nutrition "Alternate-day fasting: effects on body weight, body composition, energy metabolism"

http://ajcn.nutrition.org/content/81/1/69.full

The 5:2 diet: can it help you lose weight and live longer?

http://www.telegraph.co.uk/lifestyle/9480451/The-52-diet-can-it-help-you-lose-weight-and-live-longer.html

Fasting can help protect against brain diseases, scientists say

http://www.guardian.co.uk/society/2012/feb/18/fasting-protect-brain-diseases-scientists

Bibliography

Fuhrman, Joel, Fasting and Eating for Health, 1995

New Covent Garden Food Co, *A Soup for every day*, 2010

Shelton, Herbert M, *Fasting can save your life*, 1964

Join in

If this book has inspired you to make a success of the 5:2 Fast Diet, please leave your story as a review on amazon.com. You may just inspire others to join in too.

I'd also love to hear your feedback. You can comment on my blog at www.52recipes.co.uk (where I regularly post new recipe ideas and blog about fasting), follow me on Twitter at @52DietRecipes, or email me at j@52recipes.co.uk.

Disclaimer

The information provided in this book is designed to provide helpful information on the subjects discussed. This book is not meant to be used, nor should it be used, to diagnose or treat any medical condition. For diagnosis or treatment of any medical problem consult your own doctor.

The publisher and author are not responsible for any specific health or allergy needs that may require medical supervision and are not liable for any damages or negative consequences from any treatment, action, application or preparation, to any person reading or following the information in this book. References are provided for informational purposes only and do not constitute endorsement of any websites or other sources. Readers should be aware that the websites listed in this book may change.

Current medical opinion suggest that the benefits of fasting are unproven. Until they are proven you undertake fasting at your own risk. There are certain medical conditions that would make fasting dangerous and fasting should definitely not be undertaken if you suffer from diabetes or are pregnant or breastfeeding. This list is not authoritative and there may be other medical conditions under which you should not attempt fasting. If in doubt consult your doctor.

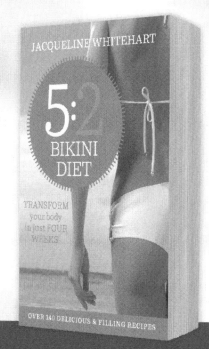

Index

29680108R00085

Made in the USA
Lexington, KY
06 February 2014